Natural Care:

70 Amazing Toxic-Free Lotions And Soaps Recipes With Simple Instructions

Table of content:

Book 2

Pure Soap Making: Beginners Guide On How To Create Your Own Natural Soap + 31 Amazing Homemade Soap Recipes...................... 83

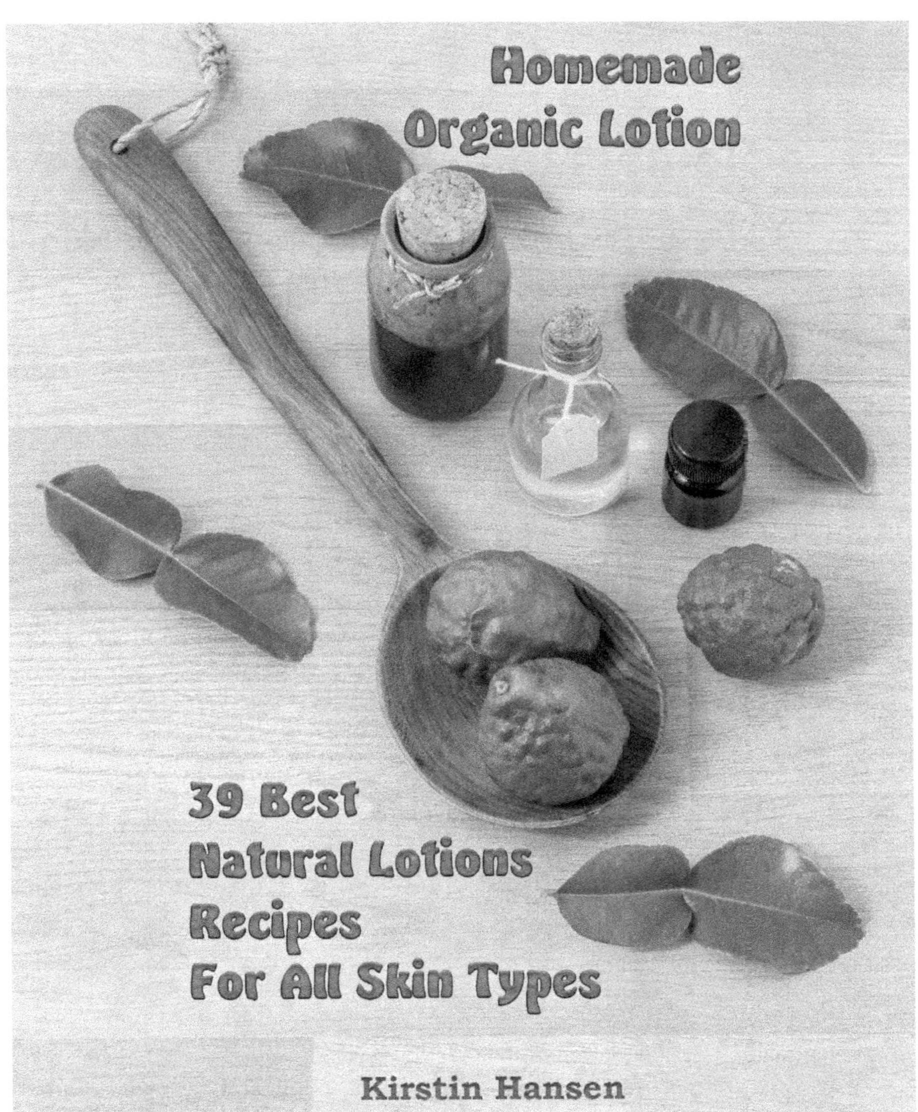

Homemade
Organic Lotion

39 Best
Natural Lotions
Recipes
For All Skin Types

Kirstin Hansen

Homemade Organic Lotion:

39 Best Natural Lotions Recipes for All Skin Types

Introduction

How much sense does it make to water a plastic tree? In my mind, not much. Most of what I've come across in the world of body lotions have been synthetic scientifically engineered chemicals.

Some people find such things to be fantastically useful advances in science. While I feel respect for what people today are able to do and create I remain in favor of a more natural approach to life.

It is a difficult market for those who share my sense of connection to an innate naturalistic method of living. Much of what is sold to us is composed of again, synthetic, man-engineered items. This is significant in the sense that often times such things are composed of individually toxic parts, yet as a whole avoid a dangerous level of toxicity.

The same can be said of products in the cosmetic industry. Frequently products contain elements which are not only insufficient at solving the problem they claim to, but are dangerous and harmful to the skin. Most of the time there are only trace amounts of these hazardous chemical compounds so the damage frequently occurs in the long run following extended use.

For the aforementioned reasons I strictly prefer natural lotions as they are composed of nonhazardous, naturally occurring substances. That is not to say that there are not harmful or poisonous substances that occur naturally in our environment. Yet when it comes to taking care of our skin it seems sensible to me to take advantage of the gentle solutions offered by the earth.

Natural body lotions have a greater success rate when it comes to fulfilling their promise. In most cases the particular skin type is not important as all skin benefits from some key vitamins and topical mixtures. There are also less cases of people having adverse reactions to natural body lotions. They do not contain alcohol, which severely dries the skin, and they maintain a soothing moisturizing factor that nourishes the skin.

Everyone is entitled to their own opinion but for those who are looking to take the best care of themselves they can, I say do it the natural way.

Chapter 1 – Before You Begin

Understanding Skin Types

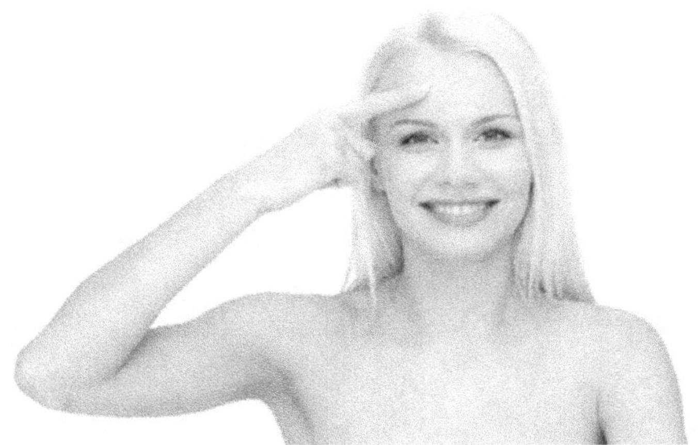

Everybody is physically unique. In your shape, size, and composition. Everything about you is unique exactly to you—including your skin. One thing about buying lotions at the store that can be difficult is trying to find one bottle of lotion that is made for your exact skin type and meets all of your skin care needs.

Not all lotions are created equally, and with the mass marketing of brands, many skin types can get over-looked. Or, if you don't have normal skin, you may end up paying an arm and a leg for specialty lotions designed for oily or dry skin and price marked way more than they are worth.

Some lotions or creams can run upward of forty dollars. What are you paying for? More often than not, you're paying for the brand name or some expensive lab-created ingredient that does exactly the same thing as its organic counterparts.

By making your own lotion at home, you can guarantee that you create a product for the skin you have, and the skin you want. This will allow you to reap the benefits of having healthy, moisturized, hydrated skin and give you the opportunity to add some protective ingredients to prevent against environmental irritation.

While every person is unique, there are several basic categories of skin types that people fall into. Typically, after puberty you should have a pretty good idea of where you fall on the scale. If you aren't sure or if you just want to double check, read through the descriptions below and find the one that fits best with how you would describe your skin.

There are four major types of skin:

- Dry
- Normal
- Combination
- Oily

Each skin type has their own traits and attributes that can help you identify which type you have. You may not have all the traits of a certain skin type, or you may find that you have some from multiple skin type descriptions. Some skin can fall into more than one type.

Read through the descriptions and if you match more than one skin type, rank them based on how many traits you have in each category. Chances are if you only have one or two traits from a single category, then it is not enough to classify you as that primary skin type.

When making your lotion, go off your primary skin type for the area of your body that you want to use the lotion on. If your face identifies as one skin type but your body is another, then you may need to make two lotions: one for your face and one for your body. That way your skin gets the best treatment based on the primary type it aligns with.

Dry skin if you suffer from dry skin you can identify this condition by the following traits:

- Small pores which are almost unnoticeable
- Red, patchy skin
- Itchy skin
- Cracked skin
- Peeling skin

Dry skin can be a result of genetics, medication, or a medical condition. Treating dry skin is important to maintain skin elasticity, comfort, and prevent other possible heath conditions.

Normal Skin Normal skin can be identified by the following traits:

- Few imperfections or blemishes
- Small pores which are barely visible
- Minimal sensitivity or no severe sensitivity

Most people will have normal skin after puberty. This has a light, healthy layer of oils that keep the skin lightly moisturized and gives a "radiant" appearance.

Combination Skin Combination skin affects the highest percentage of individuals. Combination skin means having more than one skin type.

Typically, this can be identified if you have patches of dry or oily skin and patches of normal skin. This can look like normal skin with an oily T-zone on your face, or normal skin all over with patches of dry skin on your arms, *etc.*

Traits of Combination Skin are:

- Noticeable or dilated pores
- Blackheads
- "Shiny" or an oily sheen on the skin
- Spots of red, patchy skin

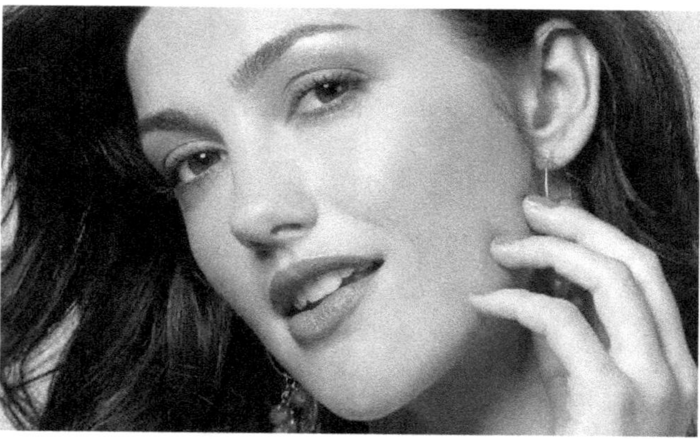

Combination skin can be treated by making two different types of lotion, or by focusing on whichever skin type is more dominant. If your skin is oilier than it is normal or dry, then focus on that skin type.

Oily Skin Oily skin is very common for individuals going through puberty and some adults. This is because the change in hormones can result in the body producing more oil for the skin.

Traits of oily skin are:

- Oversized or enlarged pores
- A thick oily sheen or "shine" to the skin
- Acne, blackheads, and clogged pores
- A feeling of "heaviness" to the skin due to the exaggerated oil production.

If you have oily skin it is important to clean your skin regularly to prevent dirt and grime from getting trapped in the pores. Hydrating the skin can help keep it healthy. Avoid drying out the skin unless you are treating on-the-spot acne. Drying out oily skin too much can result in other skin conditions.

Once you have identified the type of skin you have, it will make the process of selecting what type of lotion to make that much easier. You may find that it is best for you to make multiple lotion types for different areas of the skin.

Lightweight lotion oils: This is best if you are making a lotion for any skin type.

- Olive Oil

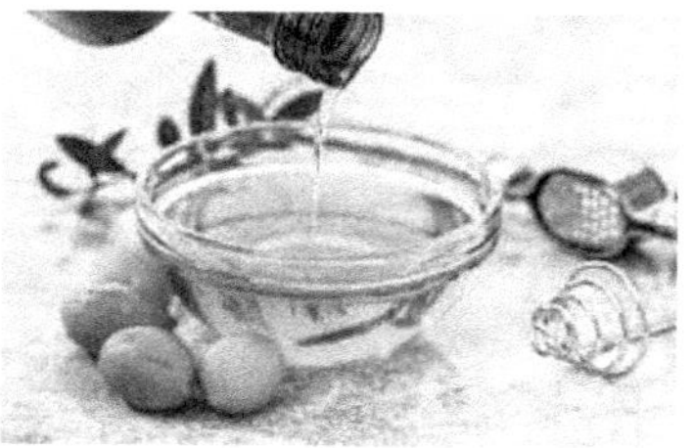

Olive oil has antioxidants and Vitamin E in it to protect your skin from premature aging, ultraviolet rays, and skin damage. It also doesn't clog pores and it enhances exfoliation to clear away dead skin cells. This is great for all skin types.

- Almond Oil

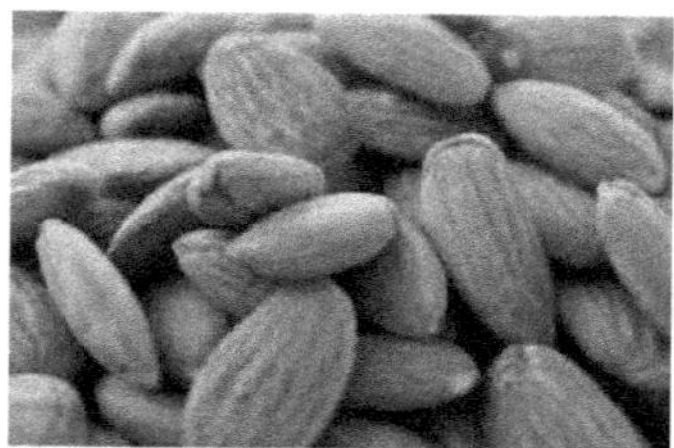

Almond oil is hypoallergenic (provided you do not have a nut allergy ;) it has Vitamin A to help clean the pores, remove dirt, and reduce acne; it can relieve irritation to the skin due to sun exposure; and it can help treat eczema. This is great for normal to dry skin.

- Coconut Oil

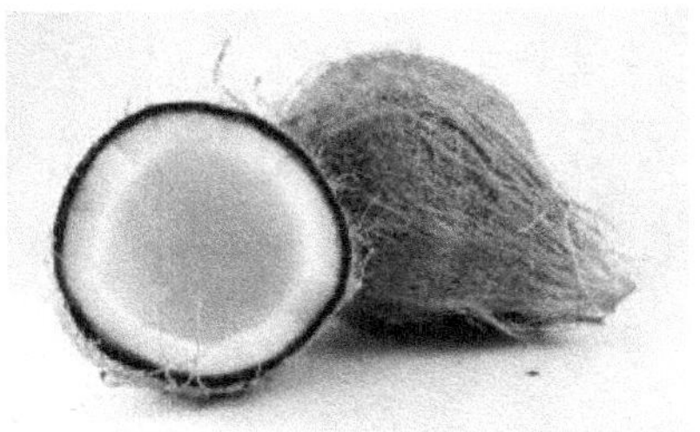

Coconut oil has saturated fats which help retain moisture in the skin. It also has Vitamin E which protects the skin from ultraviolet rays, premature aging, and skin damage. This is great for all skin types.

- Avocado Oil

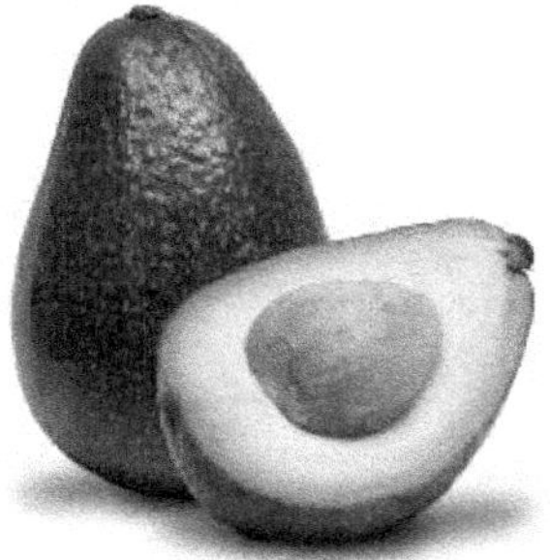

Avocado oil is high in nutrients and vitamin which are valuable to the skin. It enhances the natural ability for the skin to create collagen, which is what retains the skin's elasticity and firmness. The proteins and fats in the oil help keep the skin moisturized which can help treat eczema and other dry skin issues. This is great for normal to dry skin.

- Apricot Oil

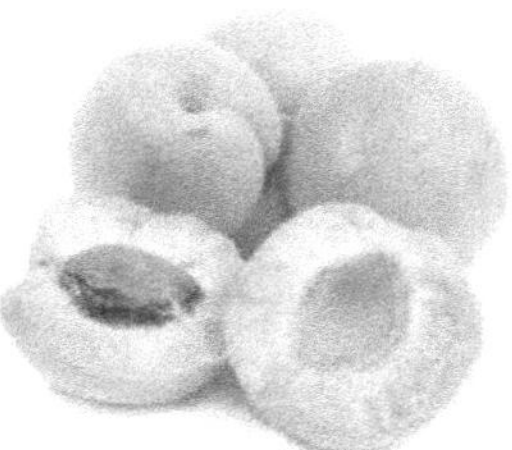

Apricot oil is great for normal skin, oily skin, and hormonal skin. It is gentle and does not leave an oily residue or coat on the skin. Because of this, it is great for the face or oily skin due to its lightness.

Heavy weight butters these are best for body butters or creams for normal to dry skin, or if you want long lasting moisture without needing to reapply.

- Cocoa Butter

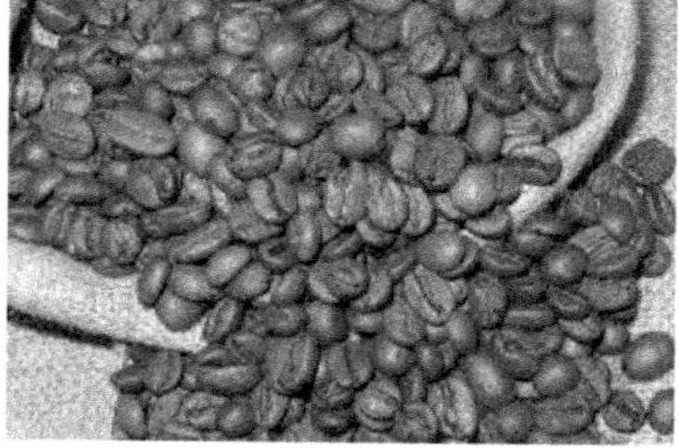

Cocoa butter is a good replacement to use if you have any nut allergies. Cocoa butter is thick, and gentle on the skin. It is pure vegetable fat harvested from the cocoa bean. The fat in cocoa butter helps the skin retain moisture and it works to smooth the skin and has anti-aging properties, as well. It is also rich in antioxidants which protect the skin from damage caused by ultraviolet rays and other external factors that can cause skin irritation or harm.

- Shea Butter

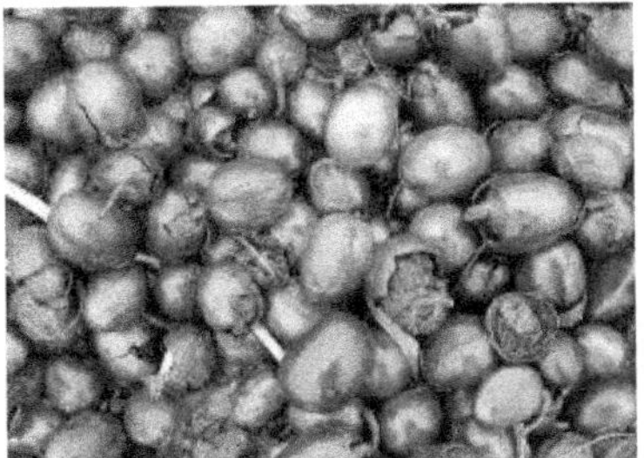

Shea butter is the most common ingredient in heavy weight body butters. Shea butter not only moisturizes skin, but the nutrients and vitamins in it help to restore collagen for skin elasticity. Shea butter also works as an anti-inflammatory for irritated skin, it reduces stretch marks, protects skin from ultraviolet rays, and is gentle enough on the skin that it can be used on babies. If you have nut allergies, don't use Shea butter, but opt for cocoa butter instead.

If you want to make a mid-weight cream, combine one of the lightweight oils with a small amount of one of the butters. This will thicken the lotion just enough to make it a cream, without adding all the weight of a body butter.

There are several different types of lotion and each one has its own function and purpose. Based on your skin type, and the needs of your skin that you're hoping your homemade organic lotion will help with, you may need to make a certain kind of lotion or several to meet a variety of needs.

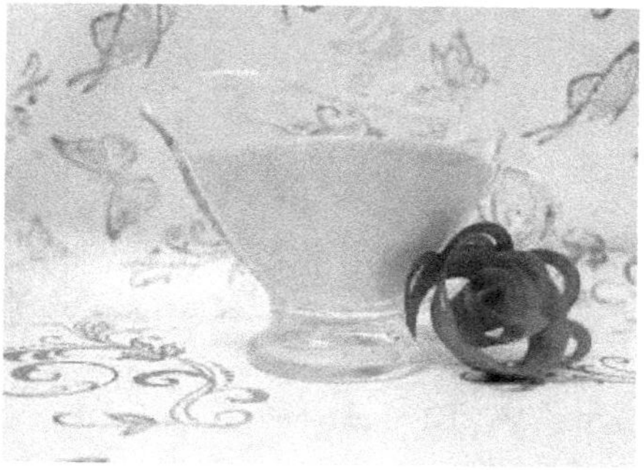

There are two main types of lotion that you can easily make at home:

- Generic lotion
- Body butter

Each type of lotion has a different function and a different base to give it a specific weight. When discussing "weight" as it pertains to a lotion, the weight corresponds with how thick the lotion is. The lighter it is, the faster it absorbs and the more likely you are going to need to reapply it. The thicker it is, the longer it will sit on the skin to moisturize it.

There are pros and cons to each weight, and those will depend on your skin type and your everyday needs.

Lightweight A lightweight lotion is going to have a light oil base and will blend easily into the skin. It will typically absorb right away, or within a few minutes. This can be nice if you can't afford oily or greasy hands or appendages, but it also means you will need to reapply more frequently.

A lightweight lotion is great for people with oily skin who do not need a lot of extra moisturizer, but still want to give their skin the extra nutrients and benefits that come with moisturizing.

Lightweight lotions are also great for hands. Lightweight lotion is good to use for your hands because if you use your hands a lot at work, and depending on what you do, you might not be able to afford oily or greasy hands which can happen if you use a lotion that is too heavy.

Lightweight lotions are also perfect to use on your face because you don't want anything too heavy that could clog your pores and lead to acne. A nice, lightweight lotion will moisturize your skin and help with the appearance of wrinkles as well as preventing breakouts. Although it is a common misconception that oil=acne, moisturized and hydrated skin can actually prevent breakouts. This is because well-moisturized skin has a healthy layer of oil which protects against dryness and dirt which can lead to clogged pores and result in acne. Too much oil can also trap dirt, which is why cleaning and washing your face regularly is important.

Mid-weight A mid-weight lotion is good for normal or combination skin. Combination skin is where you have both oily and normal or dry skin. This can result in specific spots where your skin is oilier—like an oily T-zone.

Mid-weight lotions will absorb into the skin a little more slowly than a lightweight lotion, but won't stay on the skin as long as a heavier butter. This is why having a mid-weight lotion or cream is great for the hands or body.

Heavy weight A heavy weight lotion is also known as a butter or cream. This might be more recognizable as a body butter. Heavy lotions or butter stay on the skin for long periods of time. While this can be troublesome if you have it on your hands because it will leave an oily or greasy residue for a while until it is absorbed completely into the skin, it also works the best because it lasts the longest and provides your skin with long-lasting moisture and hydration.

Body butters or heavy lotions are great for using on the body and extremities such as the arms or legs. It will go on thick and slowly absorb into the skin throughout the day or night (depending on when you put it on.) Heavy lotions or body butters are great for people with dry skin or chronic dry skin because it will provide a layer of moisture on top of the skin while it soaks in. It is also good to use for people with normal or combination skin.

Heavy lotions or butters can be too much for people with oily skin. Adding this additional moisture to already oily skin can result in a greasy feeling, a heaviness to the skin, and clogged pore which can lead to acne.

If you're not sure what skin type you have, you can test each lotion weight on a patch of skin to find out. It is recommended to test on a patch of skin on your arm where it can be easily washed if you do not like the result of the product.

The great thing about making your own lotion is that you can make it to fit your exact skin type.

More details will be provided in Chapters 3 and 4, but it is best to start with the lightweight lotion and then add more ingredients as needed to make it mid-weight (cream) or heavy weight (butter).

Chapter 2 – Lotions for Dry Skin

Pumpkin Spice Lotion

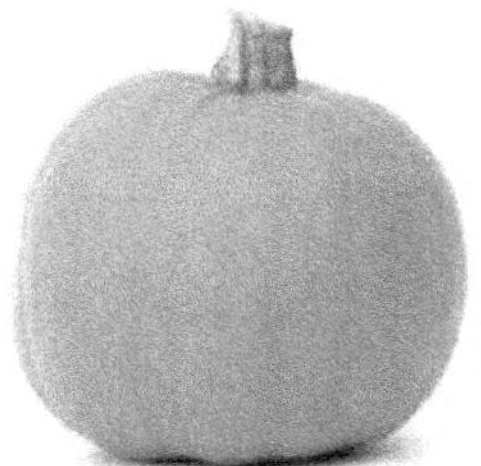

Ingredients:

- 8 ounces of shea butter
- 2 cups of coconut oil
- 20 drops of pumpkin spice essential oil

Directions:

1. Melt the coconut oil with shea butter in a double boiler then remove it from the heat while some soft chunks of butter are still visible.

2. Blend the mix with a stand mixer until it becomes smooth and creamy then add in the essential oil and blend it again.

3. Transfer the lotion into mason jars and secure their lids then allow it to cool down completely.

4. Apply this lotion to your body whenever you desire.

5. This lotion smells heavenly and softens your skin at the same time.

Creamy Coconut Aloe Vera Lotion

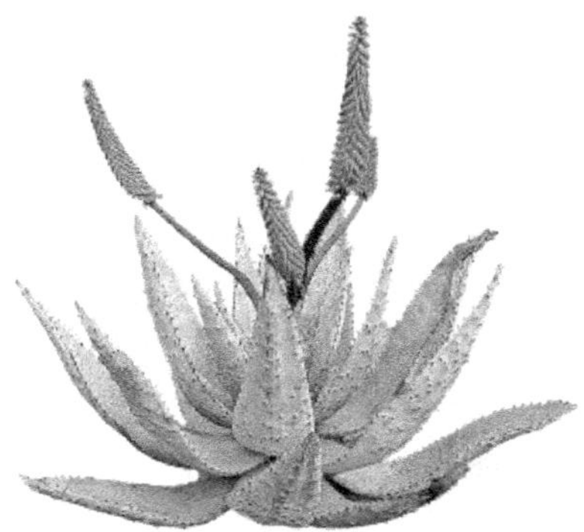

Ingredients:

- ¼ cup of solid coconut oil
- 1 teaspoon of aloe vera gel
- 3 drops of rose essential oil
- 2 drops of lavender essential oil

Directions:

1.   Beat the coconut oil using a hand mixer until it becomes creamy then stir into it the essential oil and aloe vera gel.

2.   Transfer the lotion to a mason jar and seal the lid then use it right away or refrigerate it.

3.   After an eventful day, this lotion will help you relax your sore muscles.

Creamy Jojoba Lotion

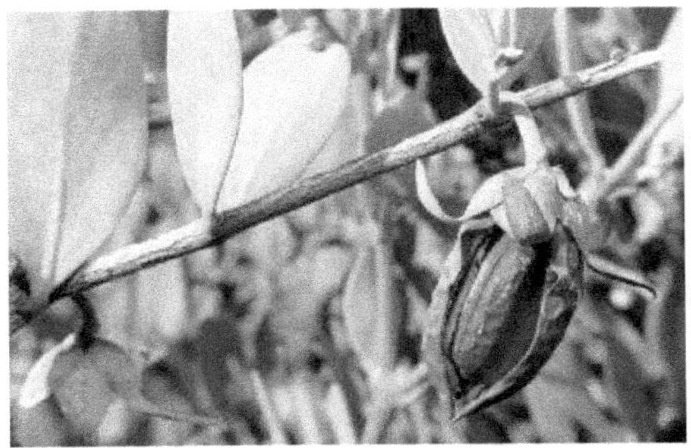

Ingredients:

- 1 cup of cold pressed coconut oil
- 1 cup of pure shea butter
- 2 tablespoons of vegetable glycerin
- 1 tablespoon of jojoba oil

Directions:

1.   Combine all the ingredients in a food processor and blend them smooth then transfer the mix to a bowl and refrigerate it until it solidifies.

2.   Once the time is up, whip the lotion with a hand mixer until it becomes creamy.

3.   Apply this lotion to your body whenever you desire.

4.   This lotion is nourishing; it will smoothen and soften your skin.

Grapefruit Body Lotion

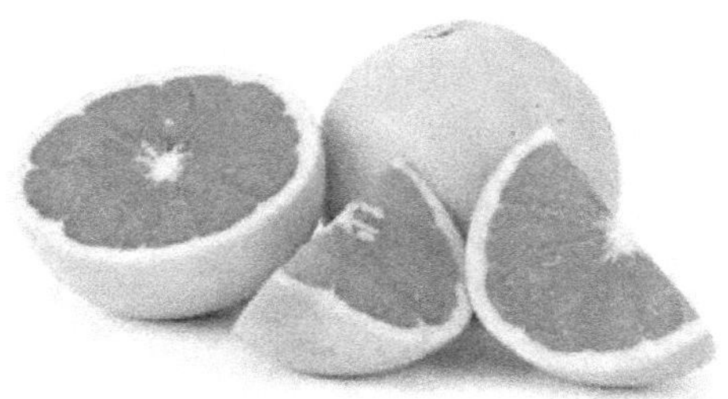

Ingredients:

- ½ cup of coconut oil
- The zest of 1 red grapefruit
- 2 tablespoons of raw shea butter
- 2 teaspoons of tapioca starch
- 2 drops of almond essential oil

Directions:

1. Combine the coconut oil with shea butter and grapefruit zest in a bowl and beat them for 30 sec on medium then turn it on high and whip it for another 4 min.

2. Once the time is up, add in the rest of the ingredients and whip them for another 30 sec.

3. Apply this lotion to your body whenever you desire.

4. This lotion will nourish and moisturize your skin.

Lavender Arrow Lotion

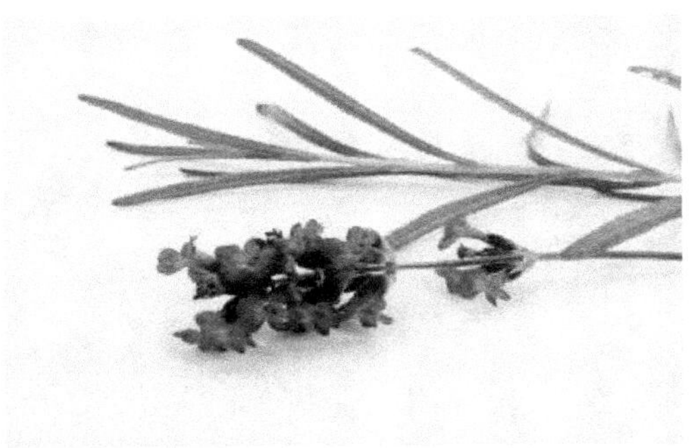

Ingredients:

- 1 cup of coconut oil
- 1 cup of raw shea butter
- 1/3 cup of arrowroot powder
- 100 drops of lavender essential oil

Directions:

1.   Combine all the ingredients in a medium bowl and whip them until their soft peaks.

2.   Transfer the mix into a mason jar and seal it then use it right away or refrigerate it until ready to use.

3.   If you want a creamy lotion that moisturizes your skin without making it greasy, this lotion is perfect for you.

Woodsy Myrrh Lotion

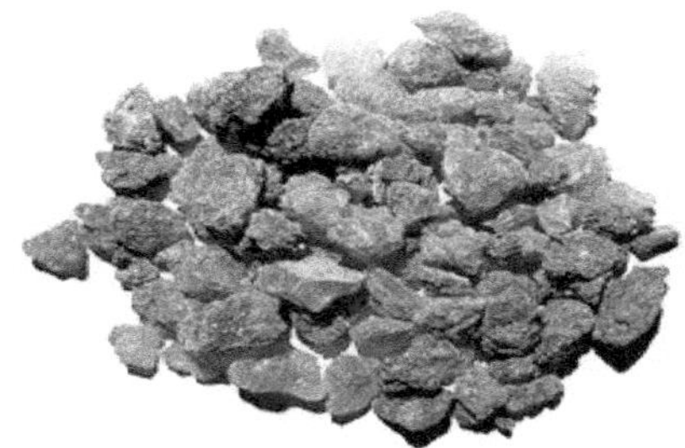

Ingredients:

- ¼ cup of coconut oil
- ¼ cup of raw shea butter
- ¼ cup of olive oil
- ¼ cup of beeswax
- 20 drops of myrrh essential oil
- 20 drops of frankincense essential oil

Directions:

1.   Combine all the ingredients in a double boiler except for the essential oils and stir them until they completely melt.

2.   Remove the mix from the heat and sit in the essential oils then whip them until they become fluffy and creamy.

3.   Transfer the mix into a mason jar and seal it then use it right away or refrigerate it until ready to use.

4.   This lotion with make your skin soft and smooth like a baby's.

Minty Aloe Vera Lotion

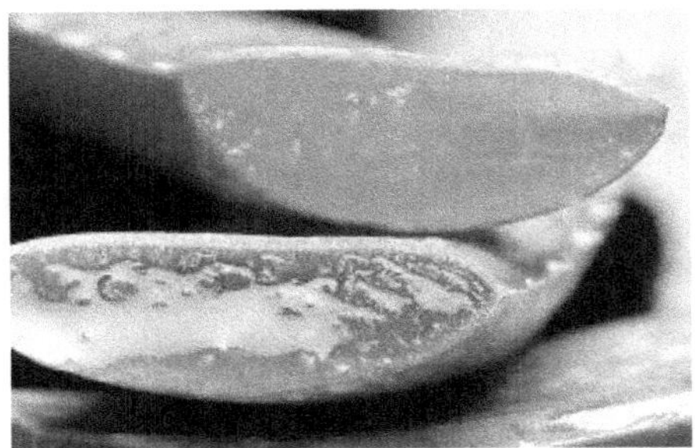

Ingredients:

- ½ cup of aloe vera gel
- ½ cup of coconut oil
- ¼ cup of beeswax, grated
- 1/8 teaspoon of peppermint oil

Directions:

1.   Melt the wax with coconut oil in a double boiler then remove it from the heat.

2.   Add in the peppermint oil with aloe vera gel and whisk them until they become smooth.

3.   Place the lotion in an ice bath and stir it until it becomes creamy and slightly thick then allow it to cool down for 1 h.

4.   Once the time is up, transfer the lotion to a food processor and blend it for 30 sec.

5.   Transfer the mix into a mason jar and seal it then use it right away or refrigerate it until ready to use.

6.   This lotion will be sooth your skin and repairs all the damage that the sun caused to it.

Floral Lotion

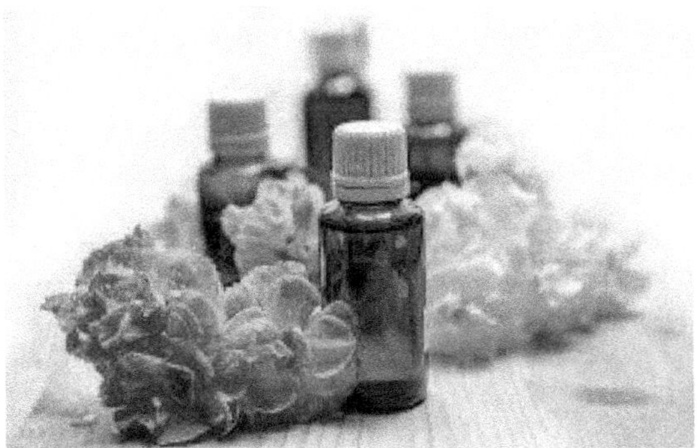

Ingredients:

- ½ cup of orange floral water
- ¾ cup of grapeseed oil
- ¼ cup of distilled water
- ½ ounce of beeswax
- 8 drops of lavender essential oil
- 8 drops of orange essential oil

Directions:

1. Melt the wax with grapeseed oil in a double boil then remove it from the heat and allow it to cool down until it becomes warm to the touch.

2.   Stir in the distilled water with orange floral water then transfer them to a food processor and blend them smoothly.

3.   Add in the essential oils to the lotion mix and blend them for 30 sec.

4.   Transfer the lotion into a mason jar and seal it then use it right away or refrigerate it until ready to use.

5.   You can use this lotion every day especially if you have dry skin, and you can use it on your babies as well.

Nutty Roses Lotion

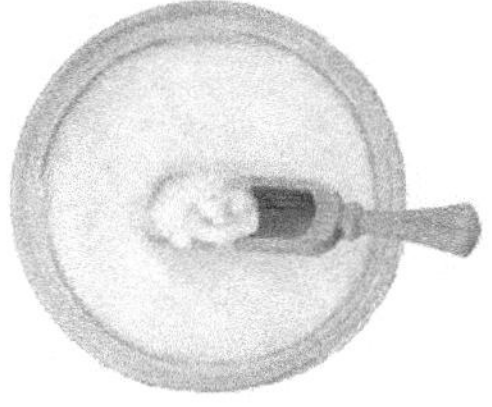

Ingredients:

- 1 cup of raw shea butter
- ½ cup of coconut oil
- ½ cup of sweet almond oil
- 5 drops of carrot seed essential oil
- 5 drops of rosemary essential oil

Directions:

1. Melt the almond oil with butter and coconut oil in a double boiler then stir in the essential oils right away.

2. Chill the lotion in the fridge for 2 h until it hardens then whip it with a hand mixer until it becomes creamy and soft.

3. Transfer the lotion into a mason jar and seal it then use it right away or refrigerate it until ready to use.

4. This lotion will keep your skin moisturized and soft the whole day.

Lavender Roses Lotion

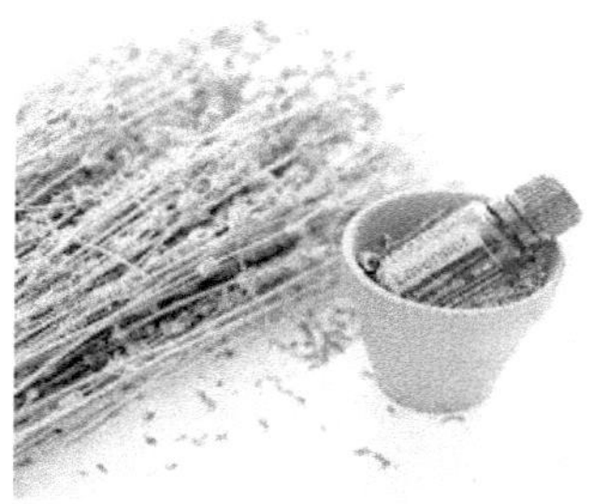

Ingredients:

- 16 ounces of baby lotion
- 8 ounces of Vitamin E cream
- 8 ounces of Vaseline
- 5 drops of rose essential oil
- 5 drops of lavender essential oil

Directions:

1. Combine all the ingredients in a mixing bowl then whip them until they become creamy.

2. Transfer the lotion into a mason jar and seal it then use it right away or refrigerate it until ready to use.

3. This is an incredible moisturizing lotion that will leave your skin smelling heavenly.

Frankincense Vanilla Lotion

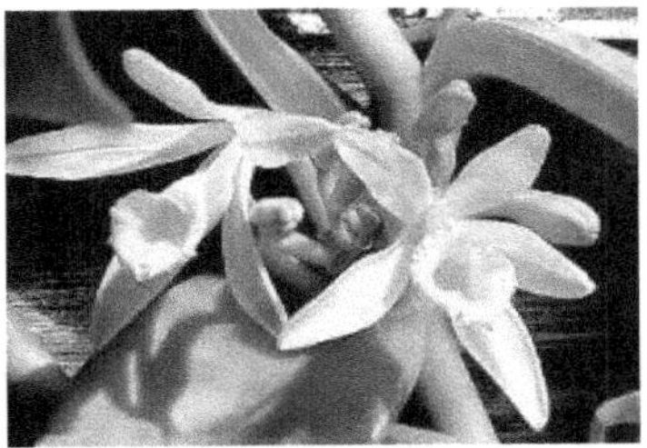

Ingredients:

- 1 cup of olive oil
- ¼ cup of beeswax
- ¼ cup of coconut oil
- 2 tablespoons of cocoa butter
- 1 teaspoon of vitamin E oil
- 5 drops of vanilla essential oil
- 5 drops of frankincense essential oil

Directions:

1. Stir all the ingredients in the bowl of a double boiler.

2. Transfer the lotion into a mason jar and seal it then use it right away or refrigerate it until ready to use.

3. This is an incredible moisturizing lotion that will leave your smelling skin heavenly.

Lavender Lemon Lotion

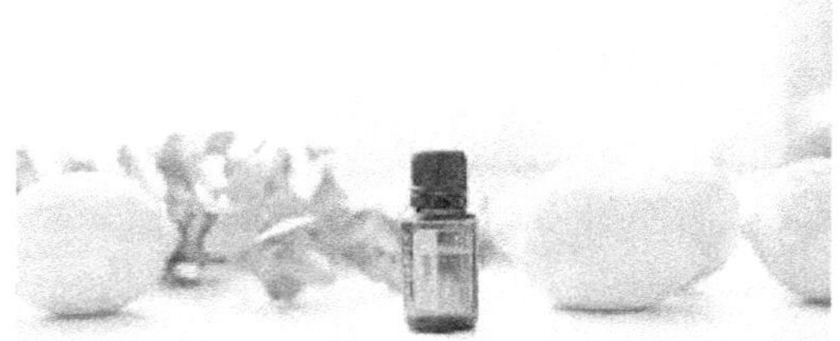

Ingredients:

- 1 cup of aloe vera gel
- ½ cup of sweet almond oil
- ½ cup of beeswax, grated
- 1 teaspoon of vitamin E oil
- 5 drops of lavender essential oil
- 5 drops of lemon essential oil
- 5 drops of Eucalyptus essential oil

Directions:

1. Whisk the aloe vera gel with vitamin E oil and almond oil in a small bowl then set it aside.

2.   Melt the beeswax in a double boiler then pour it in a food processor and add to it the oils and aloe vera mix.

3.   Cover the processor and blend them smooth then add in the essential oils and blend them again until you get a creamy mix.

4.   This lotion will repair and moisturize your skin, especially in the harsh winter.

Tea Carrot Lotion

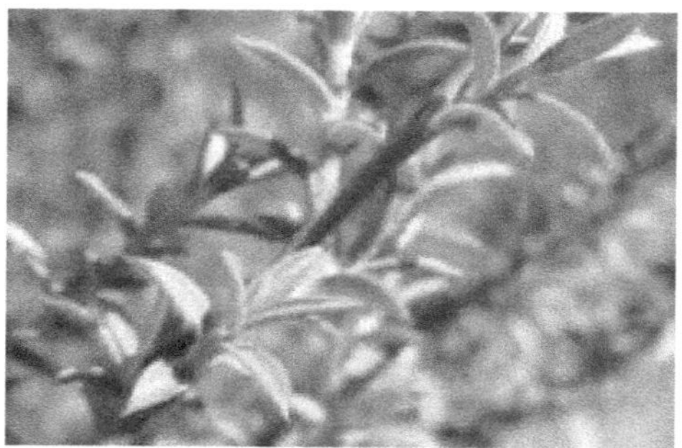

Ingredients:

- 4 ounces of shea butter
- 2 tablespoons of avocado oil
- 10 drops of lavender essential oil
- 5 drops of carrot seed oil
- 5 drops of tea tree essential oil
- 5 drops of rosemary essential oil

Directions:

1. Place the butter in a saucepan and melt it over low heat then stir into it the avocado oil and remove it from the heat.

2. Refrigerate the mix for 15 to 20 min until it starts to harden.

3.   Once the time is up, add in the essential oils to the mix and whip them until they become light and creamy.

4.   Transfer the lotion into a mason jar and seal it then use it right away or refrigerate it until ready to use.

5.   This is an incredible moisturizing lotion will nourish your skin and provide with all the vitamins that it needs.

Chamomile Lotion Bar

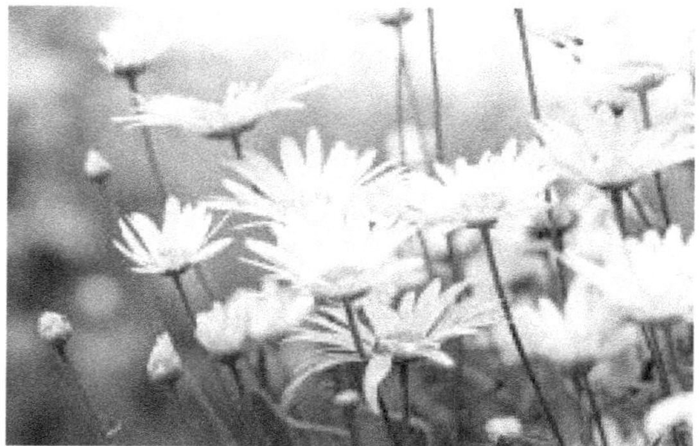

Ingredients:

- 1/8 cup of coconut oil
- 2 1/8 tablespoons of cocoa butter
- 1 1/3 tablespoon of beeswax

- 1 teaspoon of peppermint essential oil
- ½ teaspoon of lavender essential oil
- ¼ teaspoon of rosemary essential oil
- 15 drops of chamomile essential oil

Directions:

1.   Combine the beeswax with cocoa butter and coconut oil in a double boiler and stir them until they completely.

2.   Remove the oils from the heat and stir into it the essential oils.

3.   Transfer the lotion into a mason jar and seal it then use it right away or refrigerate it until ready to use.

4.   This lotion is an amazing moisturizer for your skin; ycu can use it for your baby as well without worrying about anything.

Chapter 4 – Lotions for Oily Skin

Tropical Creamy Lotion

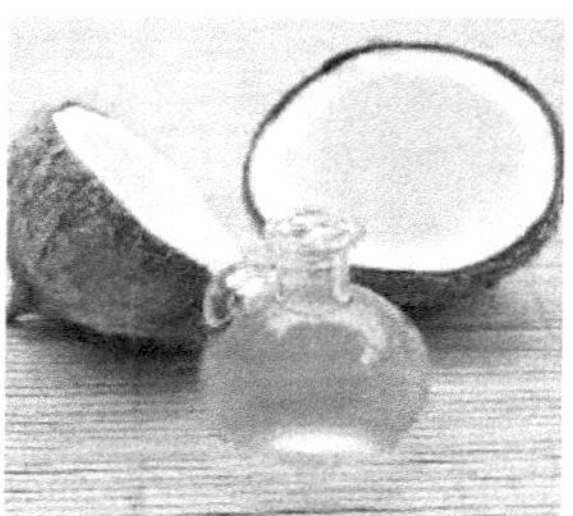

Ingredients:

- ½ cup of coconut oil
- ½ cup of shea butter
- 10 drops of orange essential oil
- 10 drops of lime essential oil
- 5 drops of grapefruit essential oil

Directions:

1.   Melt the shea butter with coconut oil in a double boiler and allow it to cool down for 3 to 5 min.

2.   Add in the essential oils and whip the mix until it becomes creamy then use it after shaving and enjoy.

3.   This lotion will make your skin so soft and fresh not to mention that it will stop the itching feeling that you get after shaving.

Bluish Winter Lotion

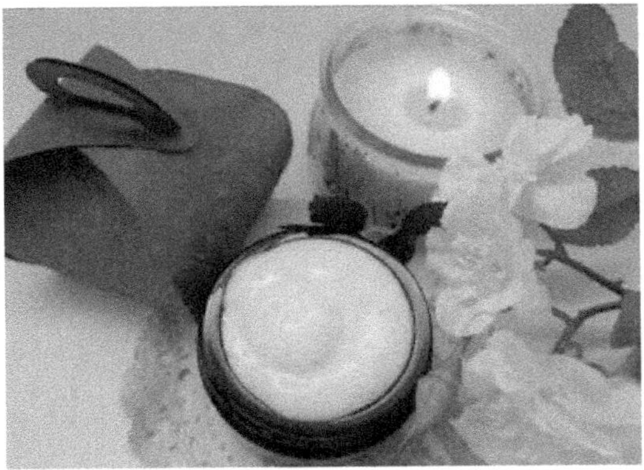

Ingredients:

- 27 ounces of baby lotion
- 8 ounces of coconut oil
- 7 ounces of Aquaphor
- 4 ounces of Fruit of Earth vitamin E cream

Directions:

1. Combine all the ingredients in a large bowl and whip them with a hand mixer until they become creamy.

2. Transfer the mix into a mason jar and refrigerate it then use it whenever you desire.

3. This lotion is perfect for the harsh winter season that leaves your skin chapped and cracked, this lotion will repair your skin and keep it moisturized.

Lavender Facial Lotion

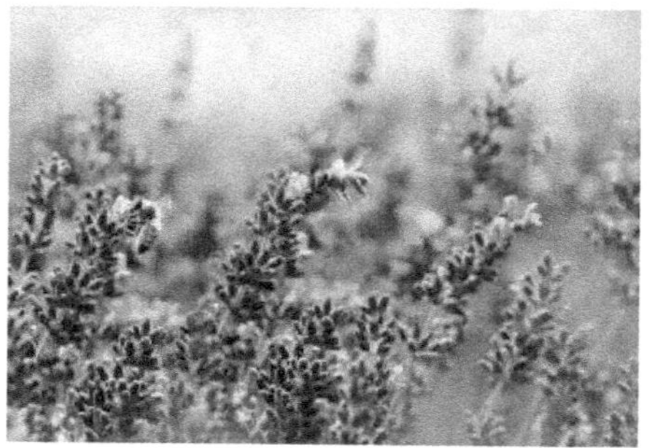

Ingredients:

- 3 ½ tablespoons of shea butter
- 3 tablespoons of ale vera gel
- 2 tablespoons of jojoba oil
- 1 teaspoon of vitamin E oil
- 4 drops of lavender essential oil

Directions:

1. Melt the jojoba oil with butter in a double boiler then stir into them the aloe vera gel and whip them until they become creamy.

2. Add in the rest of the ingredients and whip them for 1 min then transfer the lotion into a mason jar and use it whenever you desire.

3. This lotion is perfect for people that have dry skin; it will leave your skin moisturized and soft.

Creamy Magnesium Lotion

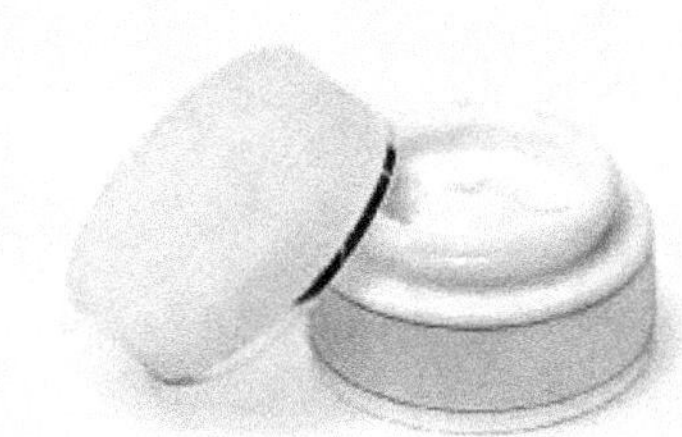

Ingredients:

- ½ cup of magnesium flakes
- ¼ cup of grapes seeds oil
- ¼ cup of coconut oil
- 3 tablespoons of distilled water
- 2 ½ tablespoons of beeswax, grated
- 1 tablespoon of shea butter
- 1 teaspoon of vitamin E oil
- 20 drops of lavender essential oil
- 10 drops of peppermint essential oil

Directions:

1.	Bring the water to a boil then remove it from the heat and stir into it the magnesium flakes until it dissolves.

2.   Combine the rest of the ingredients in a double boiler and stir them until they completely melt and whip them while adding the magnesium mix until you get a creamy mix.

3.   Transfer the lotion into a mason jar and refrigerate it then use it whenever you desire.

4.   This lotion will nourish your skin and make it healthy as well as relieve your body from all the tension and help you sleep well.

Calming Lavender Lotion

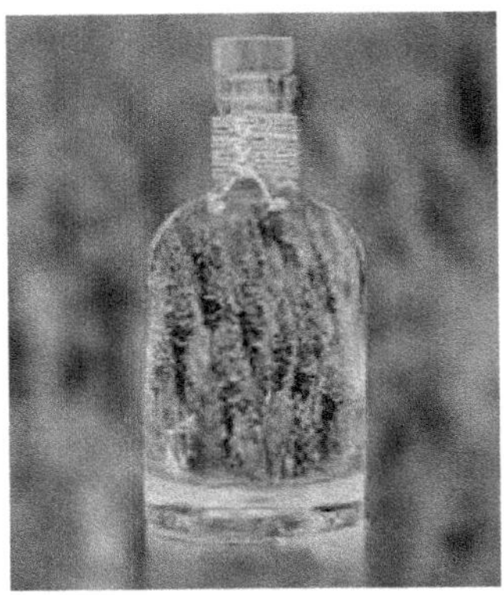

Ingredients:

- ½ cup of organic coconut oil
- 25 drops of lavender essential oil
- 25 drops of Melrose essential oil

Directions:

1. Melt the coconut oil in a double boiler then stir into it the essential oils and transfer it to a mason jar.

2. After a long tiring day, this lotion will help you relax and make you feel so good about yourself.

Rosy Shea Lotion

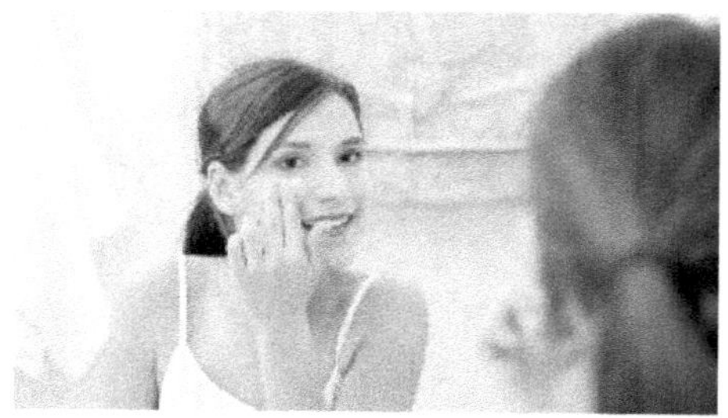

Ingredients:

- ½ cup of shea butter
- 1 tablespoon of almond oil
- 1 tablespoon of jojoba oil
- 10 drops of rosemary essential oil
- 10 drops of lavender essential oil

Directions:

1.   Melt the jojoba oil with shea butter and almond oil in a double boiler then refrigerate it for 10 to 15 min.

2.   Once the time is up, add in the essential oils and whip the mix with a hand mixer until you get a creamy mix.

3.   Transfer your lotion to a mason jar and apply it whenever needed.

4.   This lotion will moisturize your skin and prevent it from drying.

Coconut Tea Lotion

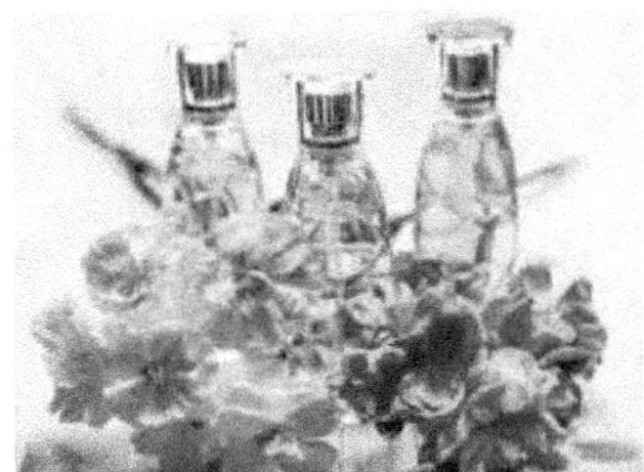

Ingredients:

- ½ cup of shea butter
- 2 tablespoons of avocado oil
- 10 drops of lavender essential oil
- 5 drops of rosemary essential oil
- 3 drops of tea tree essential oil
- 3 drops of carrot seed essential oil

Directions:

1. Melt the avocado oil with shea butter in a double boiler then refrigerate it for 10 to 15 min.

2. Once the time is up, add in the essential oils and whip the mix with a hand mixer until you get a creamy mix.

3. Transfer your lotion to a mason jar and apply it whenever needed.

4. This lotion will moisturize your skin and keep it looking glowing; you can use it on both your body and face.

Non-greasy Cocoa Lotion

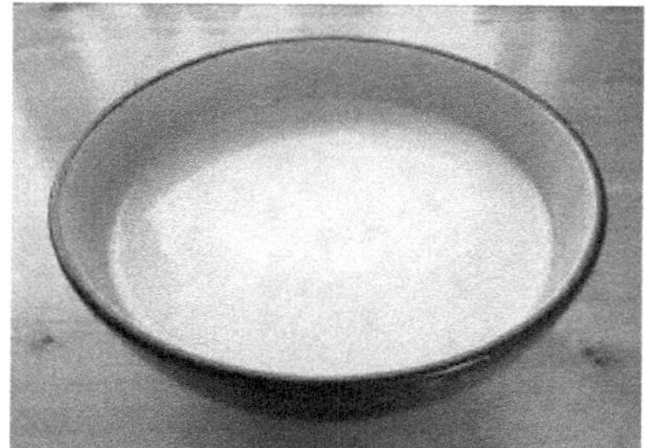

Ingredients:

- ¼ cup of coconut oil
- 1/8 cup of cocoa butter
- 1/8 cup of shea butter
- 1 tablespoon of jojoba oil
- 1 tablespoon of aloe vera juice
- 10 drops of orange essential oil

Directions:

1.   Whisk the essential oil with jojoba oil and aloe vera juice in a small bowl then set it aside.

2.   Combine the rest of the ingredients in a double boiler and melt them completely then stir in the aloe vera mix.

3.   Transfer the lotion into a mason jar and use it whenever you desire.

4.   This lotion will nourish your skin and make it soft.

Creamy Chamomile Lotion

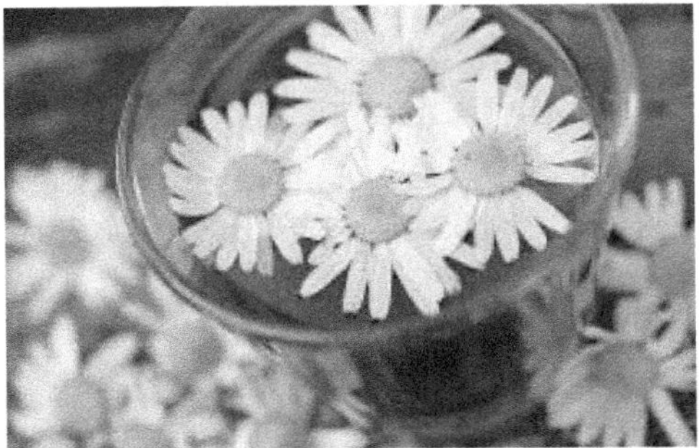

Ingredients:

- 8 ounces of distilled water
- 6 ounces of jojoba oil
- 3 ounces of coconut oil
- 1 ½ ounces of beeswax, grated
- 5 teaspoons of lavender buds
- 5 teaspoons of chamomile flowers

Directions:

1. Combine the lavender buds with jojoba oil and chamomile flowers in a double boiler then cook them for 2 h on low heat.

2. Strain the jojoba oil mix through a cheesecloth then combine it with the wax and coconut oil in another double boiler and melt them completely.

3.   Heat the water until it becomes warm to the touch and transfer it into a container then add to it a steady stream of the oils mix while whipping them with an Emerson blender until you get a smooth mix.

4.   Transfer the lotion into a mason jar then use it whenever you want.

5.   This lotion will nourish your skin and soften it as well as calm you and ease all your worries.

Minty Summer Lotion

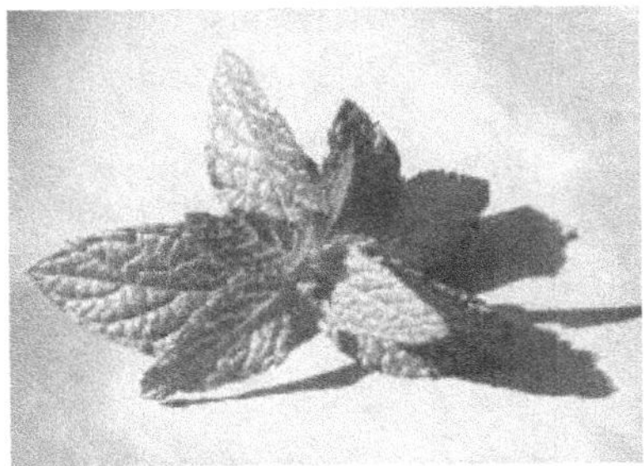

Ingredients:

- ½ cup of aloe vera gel
- ½ cup of coconut oil
- ¼ cup of beeswax, grated
- 1/8 teaspoon of peppermint essential oil

Directions:

1.   Melt the beeswax with coconut oil in a double boiler then whisk in the rest of the ingredients until they become smooth.

2.   Allow the lotion to cool down for 1 h and whisk it again then use it and enjoy.

3.   After a long tiring day in a summer time, this lotion will make you feel cool and keep your skin moisturized.

Eczema Lotion Fighter

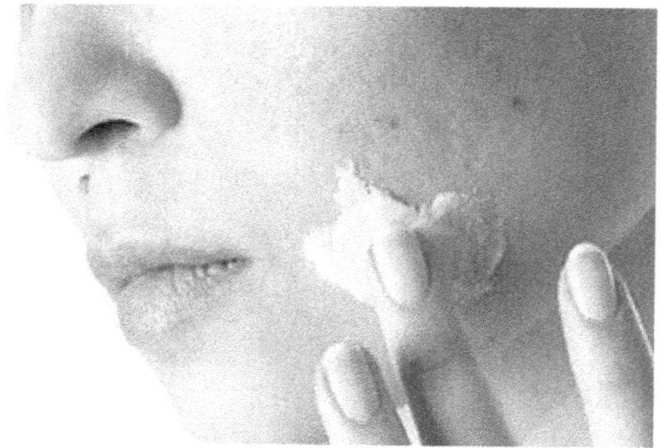

Ingredients:

- ¼ cup of coconut oil
- ¼ cup of shea butter
- 15 drops of lavender essential oil
- 5 drops of tea tree essential oil

Directions:

1.   Melt the coconut oil with shea butter in a double boiler then stir into it the essential oils.

2.   Transfer the lotion into a mason jar and refrigerate it until it hardens then use it whenever you desire and enjoy.

3.   This lotion is high in vitamins so it will contribute to healing your skin from eczema in a fast way.

Creamy Coconut Lotion

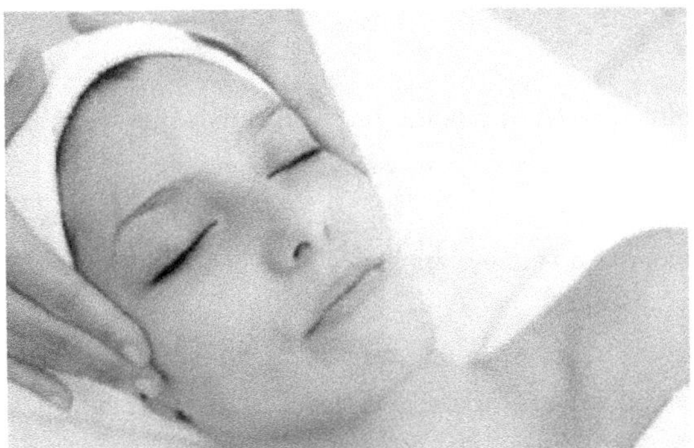

Ingredients:

- ½ cup of beeswax, grated
- ½ cup of fresh aloe vera gel
- ½ cup of distilled water
- ¼ cup of jojoba oil
- ¼ cup of coconut oil
- 1 teaspoon of rosemary extract
- 10 drops of vanilla essential oil
- 5 drops of orange essential oil

Directions:

1. Whisk the water with aloe vera gel and in a bowl and set it aside.

2.   Melt the beeswax completely in a double boiler then transfer it with coconut oil, jojoba oil vanilla essential oil, rosemary extract and blend them on the lowest setting.

3.   Add in the aloe vera mix in a steady stream to the oils mix while blending them all the time until you get a smooth and creamy mix.

4.   Transfer the lotion into a mason jar and apply it whenever you desire.

5.   This lotion is not greasy at all, apply whenever you are going it or want to go to the beach, it will keep your skin moisturized and protect it from the sun.

Historical Honey Lotion

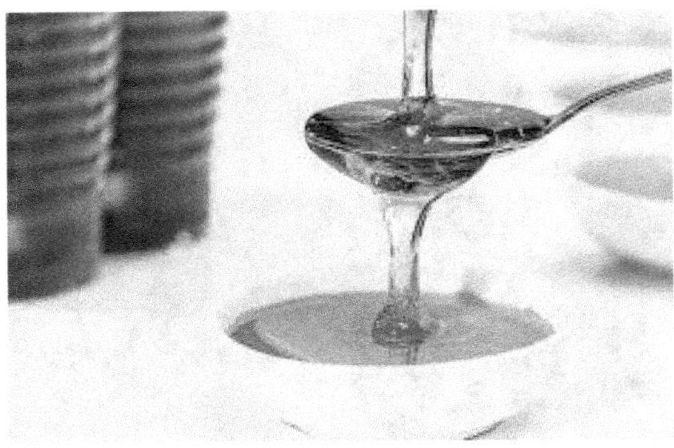

Ingredients:

- 7/8 cups of almond oil
- ½ cup of rose water
- ½ cup tablespoons of beeswax, grated
- 1 tablespoon of raw honey

Directions:

1. Melt the honey with almond oil and beeswax in a double boiler completely and allow them to cool down for few minutes.

2. Add the rose water while whisking it all the time then transfer into a mason jar and use it whenever you want.

3. The lotion will cleanse your face and keep it moisturized.

Wild Rosy Lotion

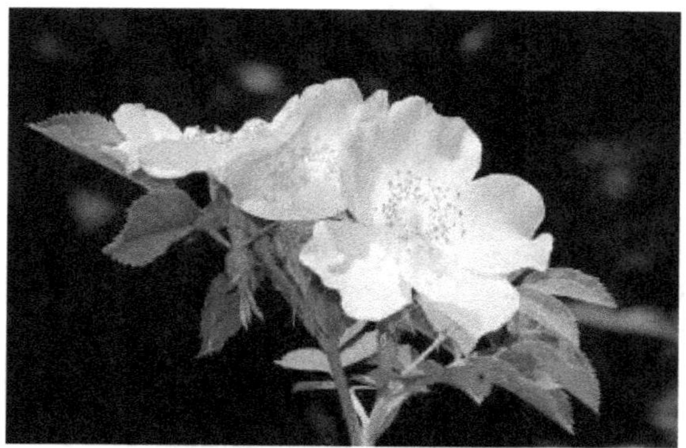

Ingredients:

- 1/3 cup of rosewater
- 1 teaspoon of sunflower oil
- ½ teaspoon of sodium lactate
- ¼ teaspoon of rice bran oil
- ¼ teaspoon of honey
- ¼ teaspoon of liquid Germall plus
- 1/8 teaspoon of cocoa butter
- 20 drops of Vitamin E oil
- 10 drops of geranium essential oil

Directions:

1. Combine the Germall plus, rose water, sodium lactate and honey in a double boiler and melt them completely.

2.   Heat the rest ingredients in a double boiler until they become warm to the touch then transfer them with the rose water to a mason jar.

3.   Whisk the mix with a coffee whisker until you get a smooth and creamy lotion then refrigerate it and use it whenever you want.

4.   This is an amazing hands lotion that will keep your hands soft and make smell good all day.

Chapter 5 – Sunscreen Lotions

Orange Summer Lotion

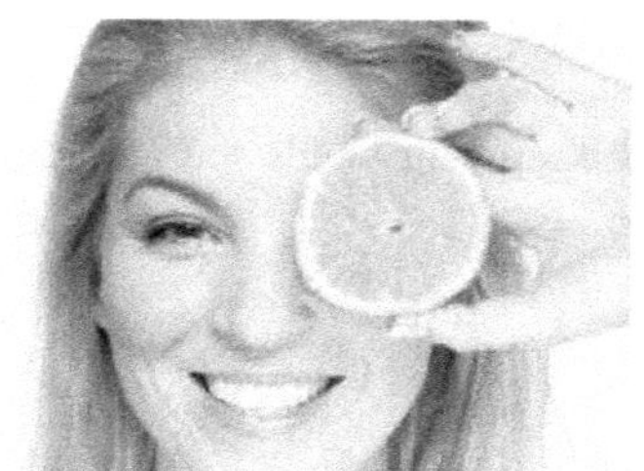

Ingredients:

- ¼ cup of cocoa butter
- 1/8 cup of sweet almond oil
- 1/8 cup of coconut oil
- 25 drops of orange essential oil

Directions:

1.   Combine the almond oil with butter and coconut oil in a double boiler and stir them until they completely melt.

2.   Remove the oils mix from the heat and stir in the essential oil.

3.   Transfer the lotion into a mason jar and allow it to cool down then use it right away or refrigerate it until ready to use.

4.   This lotion will moisturize your skin, relieve your stress and make your skin healthier.

Baby Coconut Lotion

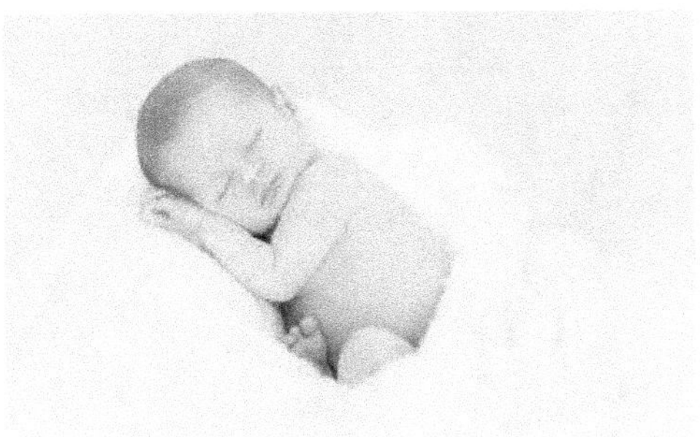

Ingredients:

- 16 ounces of baby lotion
- 8 ounces of vitamin E cream
- 8 ounces of solid coconut oil
- 4 ounces of cocoa butter

Directions:

1.   Combine all the ingredients in a medium bowl and whip them until their soft peaks.

2.   Transfer the mix into a mason jar and seal it then use it right away or refrigerate it until ready to use.

3.   This lotion with make your skin feels amazing.

Aphoristic Lotion

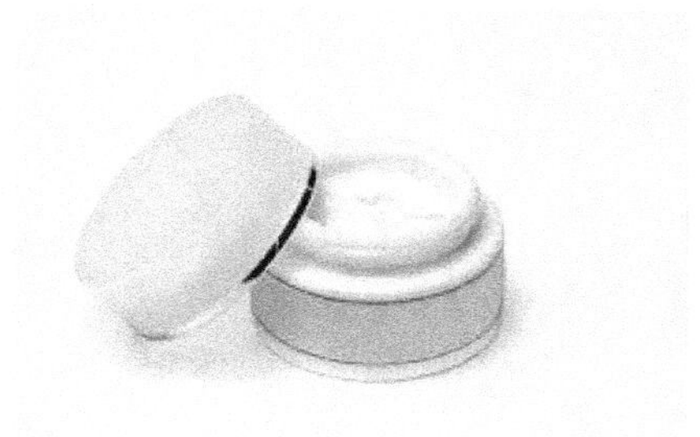

Ingredients:

- ½ cup of grapes seeds oil
- ½ cup of coconut oil
- 1 ounce of beeswax, grated
- ½ ounce of cocoa butter
- ¼ cup of rose hydrosol
- ¼ cup of aloe vera gel
- 1 tablespoon of vitamin E oil
- 1 tablespoon of rosehip seed oil
- 2 teaspoons of Aphrodite aroma oil
- 10 drops of Peru Balsam essential oil

Directions:

1. Combine the grapes seed oil with vitamin E oil, coconut oil, beeswax, cocoa butter with rosehip seed oil in a double boiler then melt them completely.

2.   Mix the aloe vera gel with Peru Balsam essential oil in another small bowl then stir them into the oils mix once they cool down and become warm to the touch.

3.   Transfer the mix into a food processor and blend them smooth until the lotion becomes thick like a medium thick pudding.

4.   Stir in the Aphrodite aroma oil into the lotion then transfer it to a mason a jar and refrigerate it or use it right away.

5.   If you want a boost of confidence, or you simply want to impress someone, this lotion will leave your skin soft as a baby's and make you smell heavenly.

Jojoba Nut Lotion

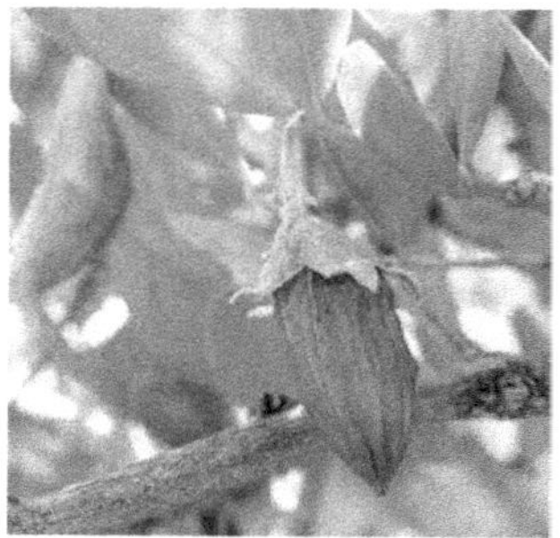

Ingredients:

* ½ cup of jojoba oil
* ½ cup of cocoa butter
* ½ cup of coconut oil

Directions:

1.   Melt the cocoa butter with jojoba oil in a double boiler then stir into them the jojoba oil and remove them from the heat.

2.   Refrigerate the lotion mix for several hours until it starts to firm then whip it with a hand mixer until it becomes creamy.

3.   Transfer the mix into a mason jar and seal it then use it right away or refrigerate it until ready to use.

4.   This lotion will knock off all your store bought lotions and become your favorite because it will moisturize the skin and soften it.

Relaxing Lavender Lotion

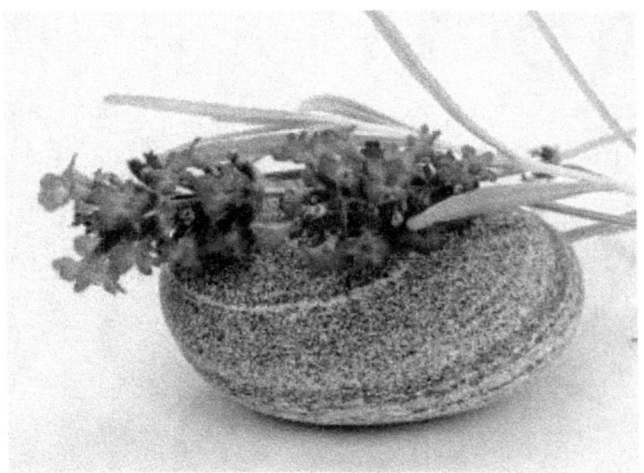

Ingredients:

- 8 ounces of distilled water
- 6 ounces of jojoba oil
- 3 ounces of solid coconut oil
- 1 ½ ounces of beeswax, grated
- 5 drops of chamomile essential oil
- 5 drops of vanilla essential oil

Directions:

1. Melt the wax with jojoba and coconut oil in a double boiler and stir them until they liquefy.

2.	Heat the water in small saucepan until it becomes warm to the touch then add to it a thin steady stream of oil while whisking all the time with a hand mixer until you get a creamy mix similar to mayonnaise.

3.	Stir in the essential oils and transfer the mix into a mason jar then seal it and use it right away or refrigerate it until ready to use.

4.	After a long tiring day, this lotion removes all the stress from your body as well as helps you relax and sleep better.

Sunny Bee Lotion

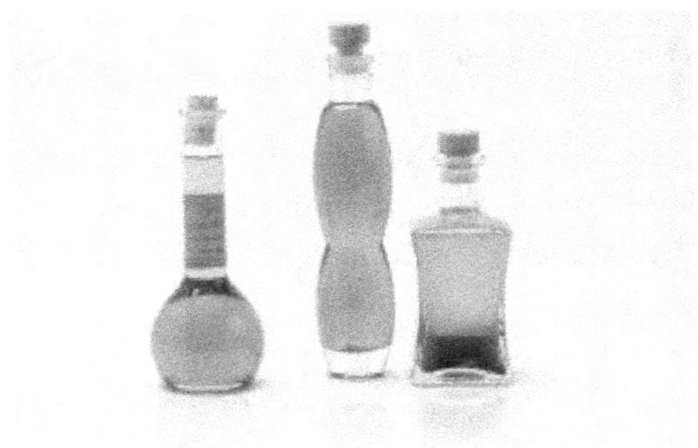

Ingredients:

- ½ cup of sunflower oil
- ¼ cup of boiled water
- 1 tablespoon of beeswax, grated
- 1/8 teaspoon of baking soda

Directions:

1. Pour the water in a small bowl and dissolve in it the baking soda.

2. Combine the wax with oil in a double boiler over low heat and stir it until it completely melts.

3.   Heat the soda and water mix until its temperature becomes similar to the oils mix temperature.

4.   Pour the soda and water mix into the oils mix in a steady stream while stirring them all the time.

5.   Allow the lotion to cool down completely while stirring it every once in a while then transfer it to a mason jar and refrigerate it until you want to use it.

6.   This lotion is great for dry skin; it moisturizes it and softens it.

Seductive Vanilla Lotion

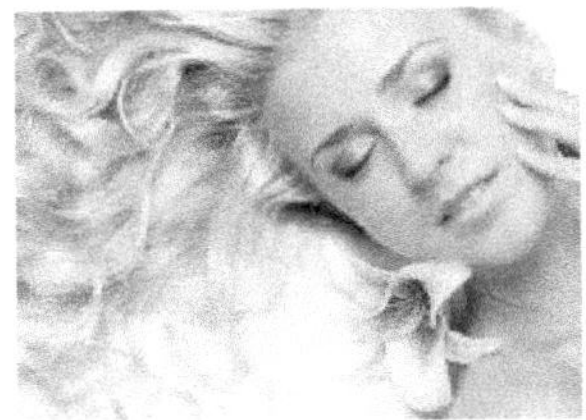

Ingredients:

- ½ cup of olive oil
- ¼ cup of beeswax, grated
- ¼ cup of coconut oil

- 2 tablespoons of cocoa butter
- 1 tablespoon of vitamin E oil
- 2 drops of vanilla extract

Directions:

1. Combine all the ingredients in a mason jar and put on the lid loosely then place it in a double boiler.

2. Stir the mix from time to time with a spoon until it completely melts then use it after taking a bath and enjoy.

3. This lotion will nourish your skin and protect it from eczema; you can use it on your baby as well.

Smooth Clay Lotion

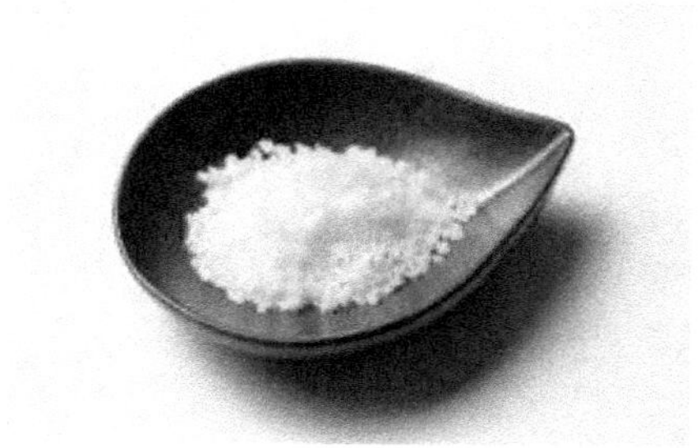

Ingredients:

- 1/8 cup of water
- 1 tablespoon of finely ground sea salt
- 1 tablespoon of baking soda
- 1 tablespoon of bentonite clay
- 1 teaspoon of glycerin

Directions:

1.	Whisk the salt with soda and clay in a small bowl then add in the water followed by the glycerin while whisking all the time until no lumps are found.

2.	Store the lotion in a container and refrigerate it then use it whenever you want and enjoy.

3.	This lotion with smoothen your skin and keeping it from drying.

Sun Blocking lotion

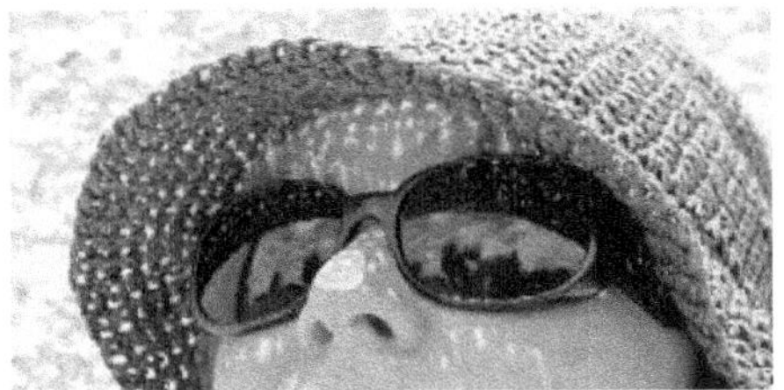

Ingredients:

- 1 ounce of beeswax, grated
- ¼ cup of olive oil
- 2 tablespoons of coconut oil
- 2 teaspoons of shea butter
- 1 teaspoon of vanilla extract

Directions:

1.   Combine the beeswax with coconut oil, butter and olive oil in a double boiler then stir them until they completely melt.

2.   Stir in the vanilla extract into the mix and pour it into a mason jar then use it whenever you want and enjoy.

3.   This lotion will make your skin smooth, protect it from the sun and leave smelling of vanilla.

Natural Sunscreen Lotion

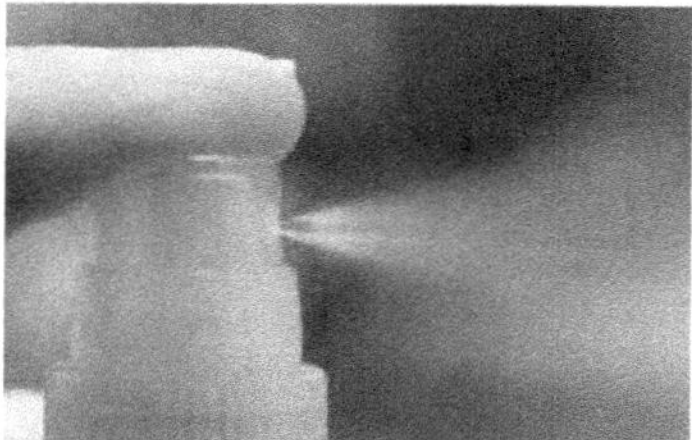

Ingredients:

- 2 ounces of avocado oil
- 2 ounces of beeswax, grated
- 2 ounces of coconut oil
- 1 ounce of shea butter
- 1 ounce of cocoa butter
- 25 drops of lavender essential oil
- 10 drops of carrot seed essential oil
- 10 drops of myrrh essential oil
- 2 drops of sandalwood essential oil

Directions:

1. Combine all the ingredients except for the essential oils in a double boiler and heat them until they melt completely.

2. Stir in the vanilla extract into the mix and pour it into a mason jar then use it whenever you want and enjoy.

3. This lotion will make your skin smooth, nourish it and protect it from the sun.

Aloe Vera Lotion

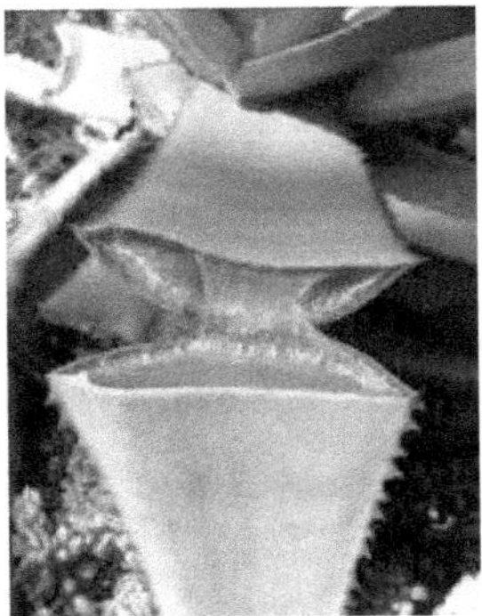

Ingredients:

- 1 cup of pure aloe vera gel
- ½ cup of sweet almond oil
- ½ cup of beeswax, grated
- 1 teaspoon of vitamin E oil
- 15 drops of jasmine essential oil

Directions:

1.   Whisk the essential oil with aloe vera and vitamin E oil in a small bowl and set it aside.

2.   Melt the almond oil with wax in a double boiler then transfer them into a food processor and allow them to cool down for few minutes.

3.   Blend the wax mix on low settings then add in the aloe vera gel gradually while blending them until you are satisfied with the consistency of the lotion.

4.   Transfer the lotion into a mason jar and apply whenever you desire.

5.   This lotion is a great moisturizer for you to use in both summer and winter.

Chapter 6 – Secrets to making natural lotions

If you're like many people who are trending toward more natural health and personal care, learning what's in your lotions and products has become more important than anything else. Here are some secrets to help you make some truly natural lotions and products so you can be sure about what it is you are putting on your skin.

#1: Choosing the Correct Plant

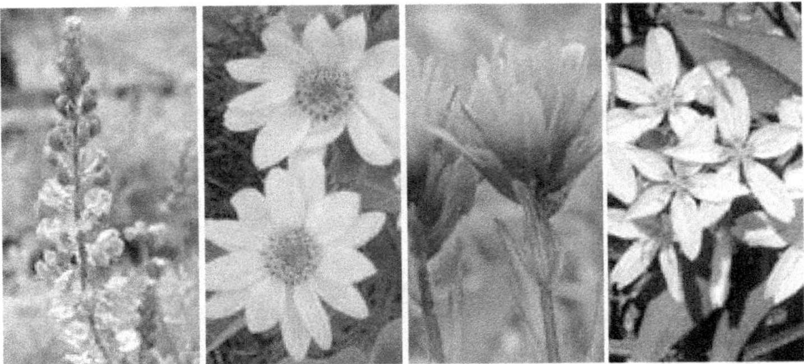

To learn how to make the finest and purest hand-crafted lotions, creams, and skin care products, you first need to know which specific plant ingredients work to balance, repair, and encourage your skin to be its best.

Whether your skin is sensitive, aging, dry, oily, or normal, nature has given us the right plant to correct the problem. Plants all have different properties. Some are astringent or hydrating, others have the ability to absorb moisture or oil, and still others contain properties that mimic human sebum, so choosing the right plant for your skin to include in your homemade lotions is essential.

#2: The Extraction Process

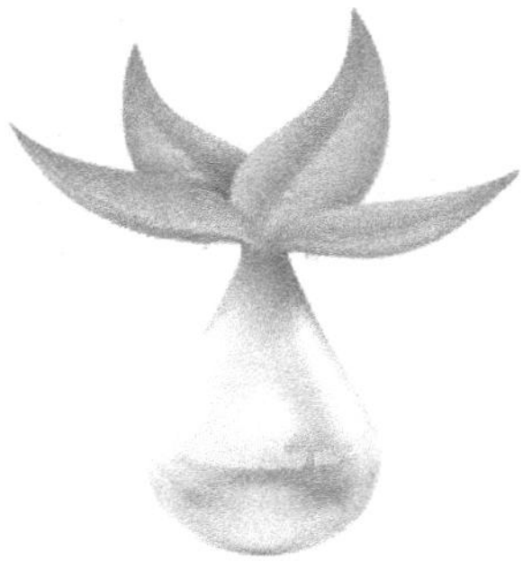

Knowing the properties of plants is the first step to making your own lotions but knowing how to correctly remove those properties from the plant - and which part of the plant to remove them from - is next. Leaves, berries, petals, stems, seeds, and nuts all contribute a specific quality.

Essential oil distillation, infusions, tinctures, decoctions, flower waters, and hydrosols are all used for different reasons in making lotions. They all require differing methods of extraction so the delicate plant properties are not destroyed.

#3: Getting the Desired Texture and Result

Getting oil and water to mix is pure chemistry, but you don't need to be a chemist to keep your lotion ingredients from separating (a process called emulsification). Different consistencies are used for different purposes and the final consistency of your product will be defined as a lotion (hand lotion, body lotion, after shave, cleanser), or a cream (foot cream, eye cream, hand cream, night cream). The result depends on your oil to water ratio and anything less than 20% water will result in an ointment.

There's a lot of information out there about how to take care of your skin and more products than you can ever imagine. Being aware of the characteristics of your skin will go a long way to helping your decide which lotions and products are best for you. Even better, to help you decide which homemade lotion or cream to make for yourself.

Importance of a natural skin lotion

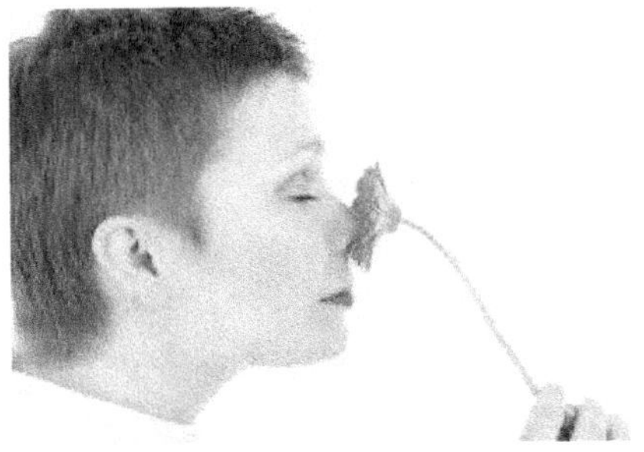

information about an effective and natural skin lotion which can penetrate deep into the skin, nourish it, hydrate it, regenerate it and rejuvenate it. It will also restore the protein balance within the skin. Let us take a look at them one by one.

1. **Nourish and moisturize the skin**- this requirement can be easily met with the natural emollients like Avocado Oil and Maracuja. They have the ability to go deep into the skin and moisturize it inside out. These ingredients have a high nutritional value which is used to nourish the skin and make it healthy from inside.

They also help in regenerating the damaged skin cells, replacing them with the new ones and thus keeping the skin soft, supple and fresh always.

2. **Restore balance among the skin proteins** - this is important to even out the degenerative reactions taking place in the body especially when you are aging. For example - with age, the production of Collagen and Elastin, which are the proteins responsible for keeping the skin smooth and elastic, goes down and hence you develop wrinkles. If you use a lotion containing Cynergy TK(TM), it can restore the level of Collagen and Elastin and make the skin smooth and wrinkle free again.

Similarly, due to the harmful UV rays from the sun, the production of the skin protein called Melanin goes up and as a result it starts depositing in the skin taking the form of age spots. If you use Extrapone Nutgrass Root, it can inhibit the over production of Melanin and thus prevent age spots from occurring.

So essentially, an ideal skin lotion should focus on - one, providing the skin with necessary nutrients to keep it healthy from within; and two, maintaining the balance of skin proteins so that you stay away from common problems like fine lines, wrinkles, age spots, dry skin etc.

If you want to look out for an effective and perfect skin lotion, make sure to check the list of ingredients that it has. It must have some or all of the powerful natural ingredients discussed above.

Conclusion

Standing in the lotion aisle at the market can be overwhelming. Not only are there hundreds of options to choose from, but if you pick up a bottle and try to decipher what it is made of it's like reading a foreign language. Too many lotions and brands use unrecognizable and unpronounceable ingredients.

Most of these ingredients are chemicals, or synthetic materials that were made in a science lab. While they won't give you any harmful diseases, they can cause skin irritation or allergic reactions. Not only that, but they can even dry your skin out more forcing you to constantly reapply and buy bottle after bottle.

If you have sensitive skin or allergies to fragrances or other allergies, trying to decipher the ingredients on the back of the lotion bottle can make the difference between a good experience and a bad one.

The easiest solution is to bypass this entire process. Make your own organic lotion or body butter and rest easy knowing exactly what is in the lotion you are putting on your skin.

Your skin is the largest organ on the body, it is important to take care of it. It is the first line of defense against the environment, and it keeps everything inside our bodies that we want to stay inside our bodies. Your skin is essential, and caring for it properly should be too.

It may seem daunting to try and make your own lotion, but it is as easy as one, two, and three. It is a less stressful solution by far to make your own lotion or body butter, than it is to go through the intense process of buying one.

Making your own lotion, body butter, or hand cream gives you the ability to meet your own specific and unique skin care needs. No one is exactly the same, and therefore no one's skin is the exact same either. Making your own lotion gives you the chance to create a moisturizer for your skin type with the ingredients that will give your skin the health and protection you want it to.

When you make your own lotion, you have the option of mixing as many or as few ingredients as you want. While the recipes above only require two oils and an optional butter, there's no reason you can't add more.

If you wanted the vitamins of Almond oil, the scent and protection of Apricot oil, and the collagen stimulus of Avocado oil, there's no reason you can't have all three. The key is to make sure that you do the math correctly so that your lotion doesn't turn into too much of a liquid and lose that lotion texture.

Some measurements for you:

Three oils:

- ¼ cup each oil for an equal dose of each.
- ½ cup primary oil, 1/8 cup for second and third oils

Four oils:

- ¼ cup primary oil, 1/8 cup for second, third, and fourth oils.

It is not recommended to add more than four oils, not only because the math gets a little trickier after that, but then the mixture might not mix as well and you risk separation.

Have the peace of mind of knowing exactly what you are putting on your body. Take care of your skin; moisturize it, repair it, heal it, and protect it. Lotion can be so much more than just a skin soother, and when you make your own you can make it that way.

Making your own lotion gives you the chance to fight against your biggest skin concerns, whether those are elasticity and collagen concerns, ultraviolet or UV rays concerns, aging and wrinkle concerns, or severe dry skin like eczema. Making your own lotion means you can make the perfect concoction to address all these issues and give yourself beautiful and healthy skin.

Don't settle for store bought lotions which can dry your skin out more or cause allergic reactions or irritation. Make your own and live life in happy, healthy skin.

Thank you again for downloading this book! I do hope you found these recipes as helpful as I did. You can never go wrong with organic and natural products, and the results will always be surprisingly incredible!!

EMMA HIGGINS

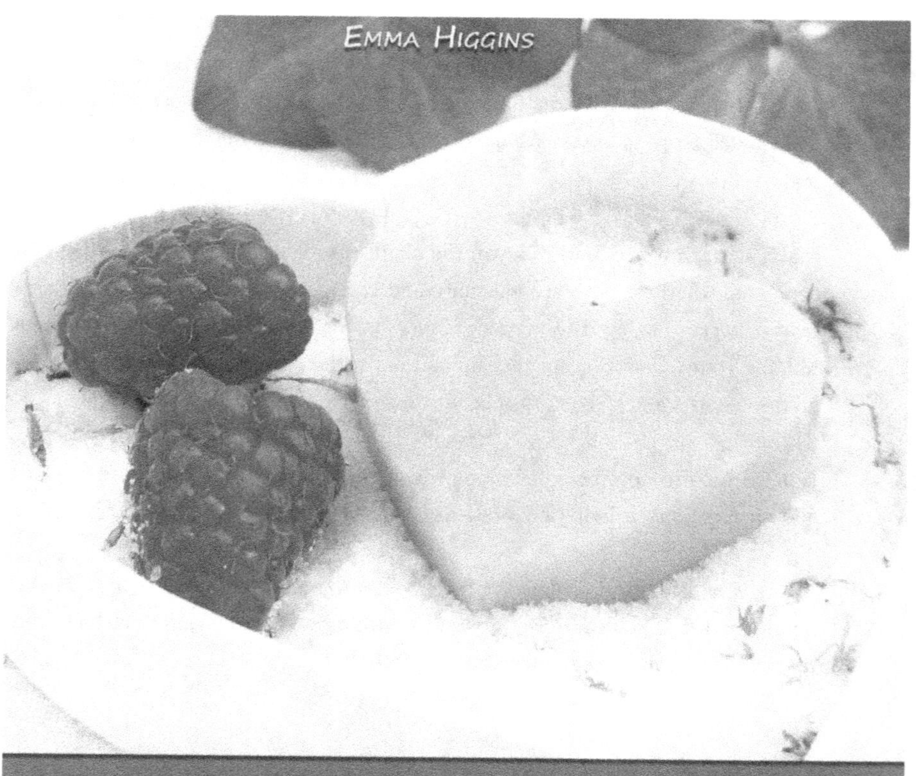

PURE SOAP MAKING

BEGINNERS GUIDE ON HOW TO CREATE YOUR OWN NATURAL SOAP
+31 AMAZING HOMEMADE SOAP RECIPES

Pure Soap Making:

Beginners Guide On How To Create Your Own Natural Soap

+ 31 Amazing Homemade Soap Recipes

Introduction

Research suggests that soap was being used as long ago as 2800 B.C. The ancient Babylonians are thought to have made soap from ashes and fat, although it is unknown as to the extent that soap was used by the general population.

There is also evidence to suggest that the Ancient Egyptians, from approximately 1500 B.C. used a soap product created by mixing fatty animal oils with salt; in effect to create a soap which would exfoliate as well! Even the Romans are known to have made a form of soap from urine!

Soap is, in effect a vital part of human history, whether washing the blood from your hands in ancient times or destroying microscopic germs; it has always been used. Of course, the more modern versions of soap have been created to leave a pleasant aroma as well as effective and gently washing the skin.

As with most products, soap was originally something that only the richest people could afford; there were very few people capable or licensed to make soap, and they guarded their skills carefully. Mainly used animal oil and parts of plants to create distinctive soaps. This ensured an elite class of customer. However, at the end of the 18th century, a Frenchman discovered a way of chemical making soap; this was the first time soap could be made on a much larger scale. This was the catalyst which drove the price of soap down and made it affordable to a much wider range of people.

This discovery was followed in the early part of the 19th century that soap could be made from glycerin, fats, and acid. This made it even cheaper to create soap and is considered to be the foundations of modern soap making; there have been no significant advancements in the science of soap making since.

The techniques and principles which were first used approximately two hundred years ago are still in use today!

Of course, modern technology has changed the understanding of soap, the ingredients are better understood and broken down which has enabled the creation of different types of soap for different situations. Laundry soap is one example of a product which is subtly different to hand soap or even bathing soaps; each has its role to fulfill. It was only in the 1970's that liquid soap became possible; it has become exceptionally popular since and helps to promote hand washing as well as minimize soap wastage.

The modern world has a dazzling array if soaps, depending upon your needs, how you wish to smell and even what type of skin you have. These constant changes, improvements, and marketing ploys help to keep soap fresh in everyone's mind; a standard bar of soap may be less popular, but the concept and use of soaps have never been so popular. There remains a thriving market for commercially created soaps; there is also a place for those who wish to create their own, homemade soap; a process which I surprisingly easy!

This book will guide you through the best method to make soap and the tools and equipment you will need to complete this task at home. It will also provide you with a selection of 31 recipes to help you practice and create your soap; you should then be able to discover and make hundreds of other types of soap!

Chapter 1 – The Need For Soap and How to Make It

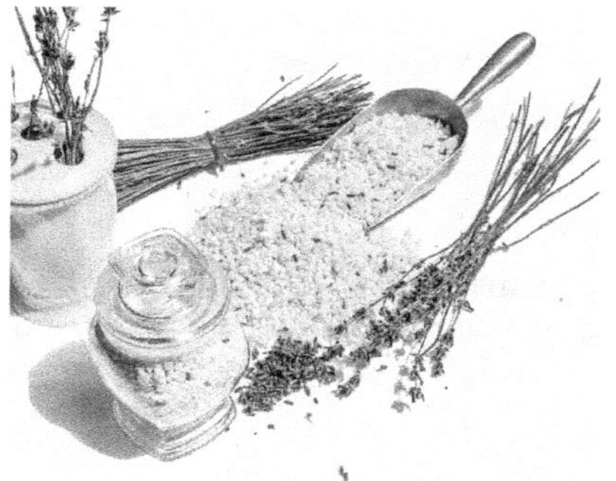

In the modern world, everyone is aware of the need for soap and its role in helping us to stay clean and healthy, although many people are unaware of how soap works and how regularly it should be used. In fact, there have been many studies on the effects of soap. There are even those who believe that soap is not necessary; the body can clean itself. There are two main uses of soap:

Odor Removal

In general, research agrees that young children, male or female do not have any odor creating regions. It is, therefore, not necessary for children to use soap to remove unpleasant body odors, although soap can still be used to aid them in smelling nice. However, adults, particularly men, do have odor producing regions. Research suggests that it is essential to soap these regions every two days unless you partake in very physical work; in which case every day is essential. Water by itself can significantly reduce the presence if body odor, but will not eliminate it.

Deodorant will always be needed to assist with reducing and containing odors, the regularity of application will be directly related to the physical duties undertaken. Washing in water will help to reduce body odor but it is more effective when mixed with soap.

Cleanliness

Soap has always been acknowledged as a way to remove dirt and germs from your hands; this is via a process of friction and agitation; in fact, modern soaps have small particles added to them to aid with dirt removal and the removal of excess skin.

The abrasive nature of these products will help to leave your skin fresh and glowing and will often help to keep skin conditions at bay. This is because many soap products are becoming more technologically advanced and can offer deep-pore washes.

It is the amount of science behind the soap that often worries people regarding what they are putting on their face or body. This is one of the main reasons people start to make their soap; knowing which ingredients have been placed into a bar means you know what you are putting on your body.

The basic process of making any soap is surprisingly simple, in fact, the most important question you will need to ask yourself is whether you wish to handle Lye yourself or not. Lye is a natural product, also known as Sodium Hydroxide. It is an alkali and can be dangerous; it is capable of making a hole in your fabrics and can burn your skin. However, as long as you handle it with care there will be no issue using it; it is worth noting that you should always use the crystal version of Lye when making salt and it must always be added to the water, not the water to it.

This lye, added in the right quantities to plain water can then be mixed with a variety of different oil. The mixture bonds together to create soap; the main difference between recipes is the additional flavorings and the type of oil used. Every oil has its own specific relationship to lye and must be used in the right quantities.

If the thought of handling lye is too daunting for you at first, then you can purchase a melt and pour soap which is ready to use. As its name suggests, you simply melt it, add your own flavors and pour it into the molds.

Chapter 2 – Cold Processed Soaps

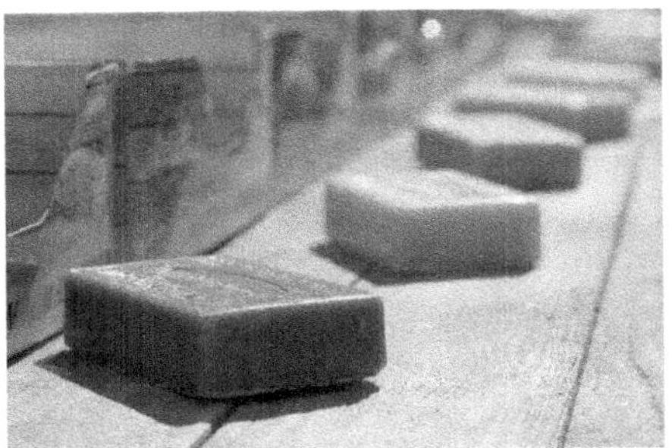

What you will soon discover is that it is entirely possible for you to create your soap recipes from scratch. All you need is a few simple guidelines, and you can formulate your blends using your favorite oils and additives. In this section, we have provided for you three basic soap formulas that you can build off of and modify if you choose to once you feel comfortable. You can create almost any soap you desire from these fundamental methods. Following the basic recipes, you will find a selection of solvents that are crafted for different uses and preferences. Each one has in some way been built off of one of the basic recipes. You can craft amazing soaps with one of these recipes, or use them as inspiration to create your special formula bars.

Basic Vegetable Soap

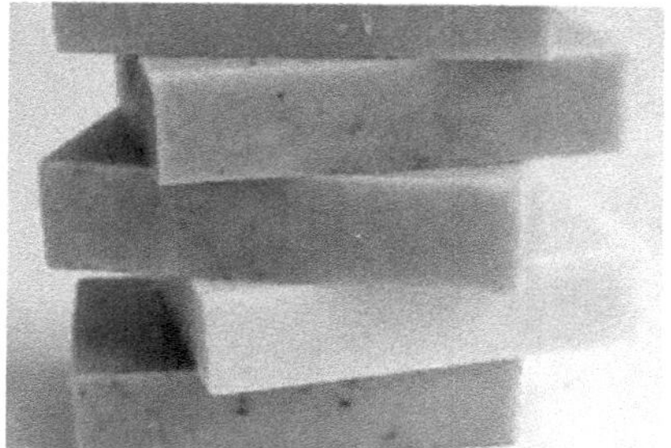

This base recipe is designed to give you everything you want in a bar soap. The latter is rich, and it is mild and conditioning. A perfect bar for every skin type including very sensitive skin. Yields 15-20 five-ounce bars of soap.

Ingredients:

- 250g coconut oil
- 500g palm oil
- 500g olive oil
- 380g distilled water
- 186.25g lye

Directions:

1. Follow the instructions for making cold processed soaps.

2. Insulate for twenty-four hours and check every day for hardness. When the soap is firm, remove from the molds and allow curing for at least two weeks before using.

No Palm Vegetable Soap

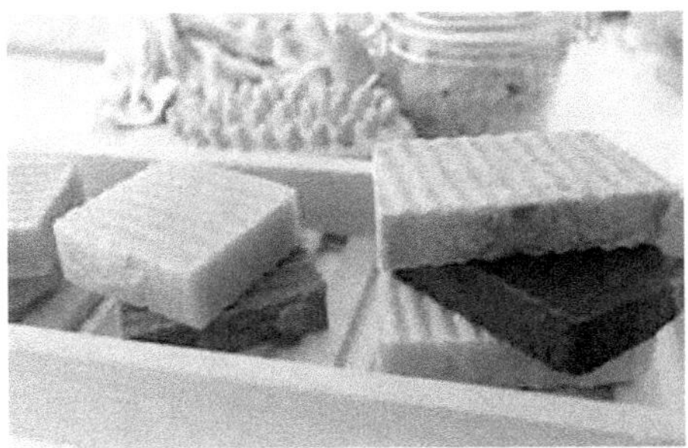

This is a great long-lasting, all-purpose soap for people who prefer to not use palm oil for environmental concerns. It can be used for skin care as well as household cleaning purposes. Yields 15-20 five-ounce bars of soap.

Ingredients:

- 250g coconut oil
- 500g olive oil
- 600g vegetable shortening
- 400g distilled water
- 197g lye

Directions:

1. Follow the instructions for making cold processed soaps.

2. Insulate for twenty-four hours and check every day for hardness. When the soap is firm, remove from the molds and allow to cure for at least two weeks before using. As you are starting out, it is a good idea to include

Basic Animal Fat Soap

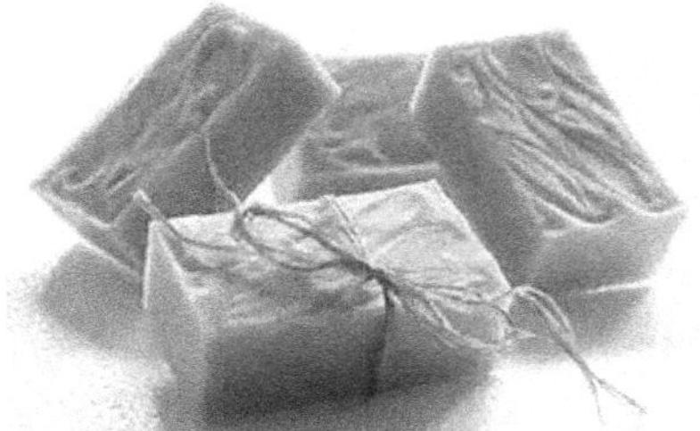

This is the longest lasting, firmest, and mildest bar among the basic formulas. People with sensitive skin will find animal fat soaps to be the least irritating of soap formulas. This particular bar produces a mild, milky, and conditioning lather that can be used everywhere from the shower to the kitchen and even in the laundry room. Yields 15-20 five-ounce bars of soap.

Ingredients:

- 500g beef tallow
- 700g lard
- 350g distilled water
- 168g lye

Directions:

1. Follow the instructions for making cold processed soaps.

2. Insulate for twenty-four hours and check every day for hardness. When the soap is firm, remove from the molds and allow to cure for at least two weeks before using.

Kitchen and Bath Hand Soap

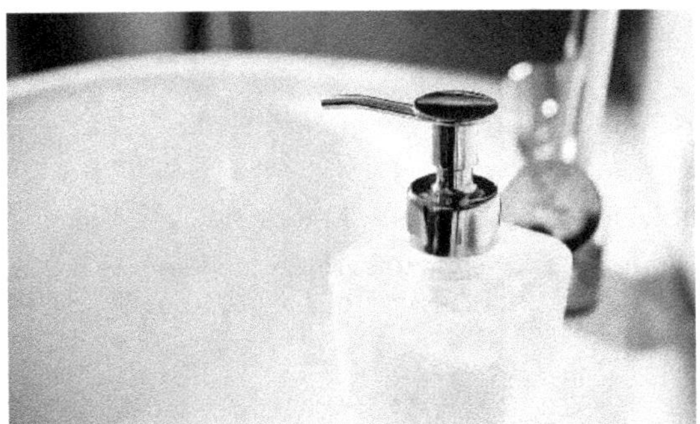

This big lathering soap contains beeswax and olive oil to keep skin soft and smooth while the brewed coffee added works as an odor eliminator that is perfect for removing string food smells from your hands. Yields 15-20 five-ounce bars of soap.

Ingredients:

- 250g coconut oil
- 500g palm oil
- 600g olive oil
- 150g castor oil
- 50g beeswax
- 440g cold brewed coffee made with distilled water
- 219g lye

Directions:

1. Follow the instructions for making cold processed soaps.

2. Add the beeswax when the soap traces.

3. Insulate for twenty-four hours and check every day for hardness. When the soap is firm, remove from the molds and allow to cure for at least two weeks before using.

Soothing Face Soap

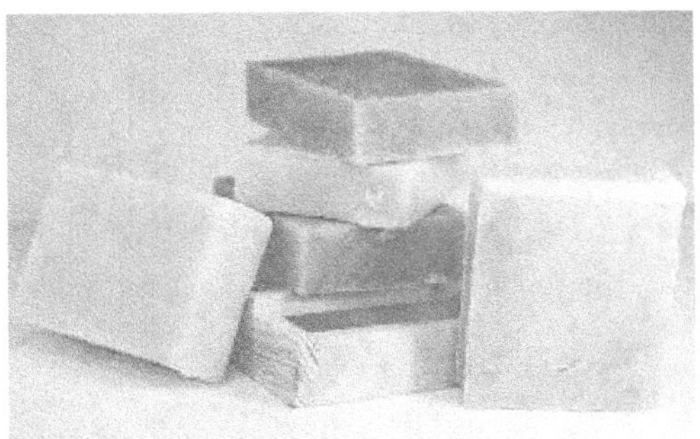

With tallow as a base, this soap is a gentle soap to use on the delicate facial skin. Shea butter, oatmeal, and lavender add additional soothing and softening properties to this mildly scented and therapeutic bar. Yields 15-20 five-ounce bars of soap.

Ingredients:

- 300g beef tallow
- 350g olive oil
- 70g castor oil
- 100g shea butter
- 50g ground oatmeal
- 25g dried lavender, finely ground
- 225g distilled water
- 111g lye

Directions:

1. Follow the instructions for making cold processed soaps.

2. Add the dried lavender and oatmeal when the soap traces.

3.   Insulate for twenty-four hours and check every day for hardness. When the soap is firm, remove from the molds and allow to cure for at least two weeks before using.

All-Purpose Shower and Bath Bar

This soap produces a nice strong, thick lather while the goat's milk and shea butter are extra moisturizing. This bar is perfect for use on the entire body including the face, hair, and even as an in-shower shave bar. The Earl Grey tea infused offers a delicate scent and light color to the bar. Yields 15-20 five-ounce bars of soap.

Ingredients:

- 300g coconut oil
- 300g palm oil
- 550g olive oil
- 150g castor oil
- 100g shea butter
- 25g dried lavender, finely ground
- 2 ounces lavender essential oil
- 6 ounces goat's milk
- 1-ounce earl grey tea
- 412g distilled water
- 206g lye

Directions:

1. Steep the Earl Grey tea in 22.0g of the included distilled water.

2. The goat's milk should be chilled to a slush consistency.

3. Follow the instructions for making cold processed soaps.

4. Add the goat's milk to the oils once the oils reach 110°F/43°C.

5. The Earl Grey tea, ground lavender, and lavender essential oil are added at trace.

6. Insulate for twenty-four hours and check every day for hardness. When the soap is firm, remove from the molds and allow to cure for at least two weeks before using.

Basic Face and Shave Bar

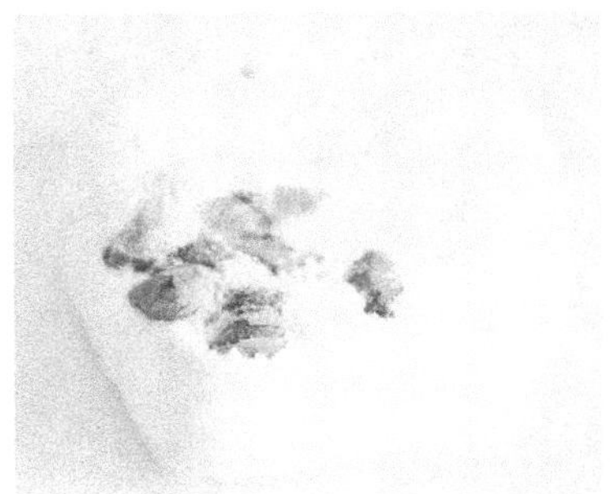

This face and shave bar produces a good lather while the castor oil adds extra glycerin to the soap. This combined with the glide provided by the clay and the repairing and moisturizing properties of the beeswax and shea butter makes a rich, moisturizing soap that will leave your face and body soothed, even after a shave. Yields 15-20 five-ounce bars of soap.

Ingredients:

- 200g coconut oil
- 300g vegetable shortening
- 400g olive oil
- 150g castor oil
- 40g bentonite clay (added at trace)
- 25g beeswax
- 100g shea butter
- 336g distilled water
- 167g lye

Directions:

1.   Follow the instructions for making cold processed soaps.

2.   Insulate for twenty-four hours and check every day for hardness. When the soap is firm, remove from the molds and allow to cure for at least two weeks before using.

Masculine Face and Shave Bar

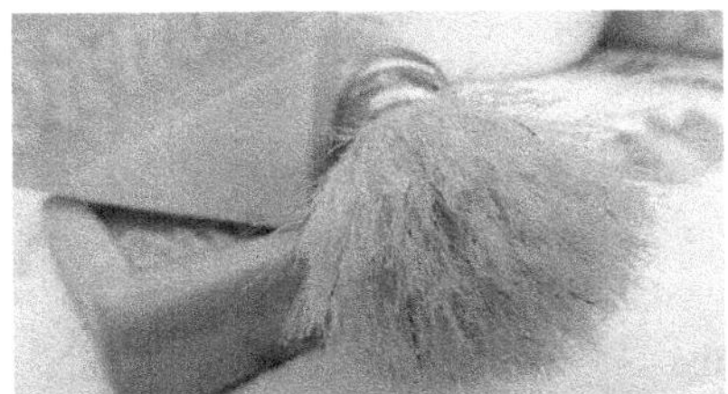

A shave bar created specifically for men, the coconut oil, castor oil and the IPA produces a big thick lather. The hemp oil provides a light, nutty oil but also offers a moisturizing and repairing component that is rich in vitamins and healing to the skin. The clay adds a glide that allows your shaver to slide smoothly over the skin. The hops are softening to facial hair and also have antibacterial properties, so it acts preventatively in healing any tiny nicks or abrasions that may occur. Yields 15-20 five-ounce bars of soap.

Ingredients:

- 300g beef tallow
- 300g olive oil
- 150g coconut oil
- 150g castor oil
- 200g hemp oil
- 100g shea butter
- 25g liquid vitamin e
- 50g bentonite clay
- 25g fresh ground hops
- 342g IPA (beer)
- 170g lye

Directions:

In this formula, the beer replaces the water. For best results, a day or two before making the soap, pour the beer into a large mason jar. A couple of times a day, shake the jar, and once the foam settles, open it slowly and remove the lid for thirty minutes to an hour. It will eliminate the carbonation in the beer. Too much carbonation can be a hazard during the soap making process, so it is best to remove it as much as possible. Some soap makers prefer to cook off the alcohol in the beer, which will also lessen the carbonation, however, this is not necessary as long as you are using a beer that is of typical alcohol content.

1.   Follow the instructions for making cold processed soaps.

2.   Add the vitamin E, bentonite clay and hops trace.

3.   Insulate for twenty-four hours and check every day for hardness. When the soap is firm, remove from the molds and allow to cure for at least two weeks before using.

Country Pantry Soap

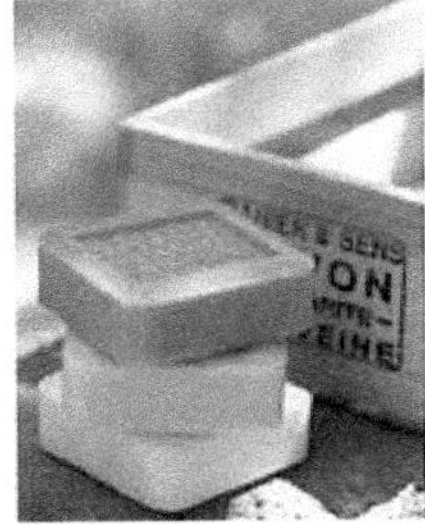

A simple, basic soap made from most oils that you would find in any small grocery store or country pantry. Nothing fancy here and no outside suppliers needed. These oils produce a nice, conditioning bar of soap. Yields 15-20 five-ounce bars of soap.

Ingredients:

- 850g lard
- 250g corn oil
- 500g olive oil
- 250g canola oil
- 506g distilled water
- 252g lye

Directions:

1. Follow the instructions for making cold processed soaps.

2. Insulate for twenty-four hours and check every day for hardness. When the soap is firm, remove from the molds and allow to cure for at least two weeks before using.

City Pantry Soap

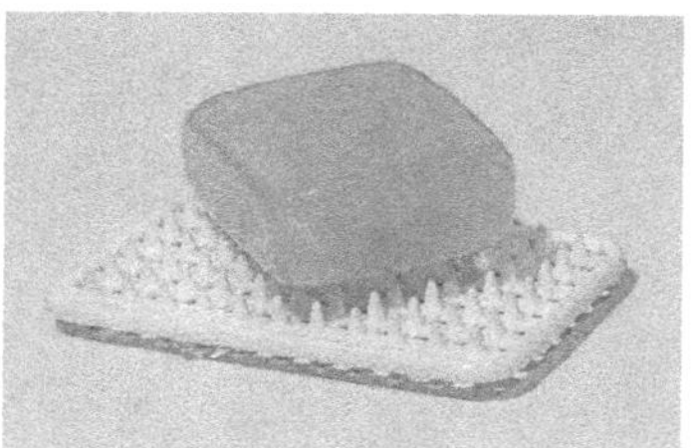

Much like the Country Pantry Soap, the City Pantry Soap shows you how you can make a perfect, all-purpose bar of soap from ingredients that are inexpensive and easy to find with a single trip to your supermarket. Yields 15-20 five-ounce bars of soap.

Ingredients:

* 250g coconut oil
* 300g olive oil
* 250g soya bean oil
* 400g vegetable shortening
* 356g distilled water
* 177g lye

Directions:

1. Follow the instructions for making cold processed soaps.

2. Insulate for twenty-four hours and check every day for hardness. When the solvent is firm, remove from the molds and allow to cure for at least two weeks before using.

Winter Facial Bar

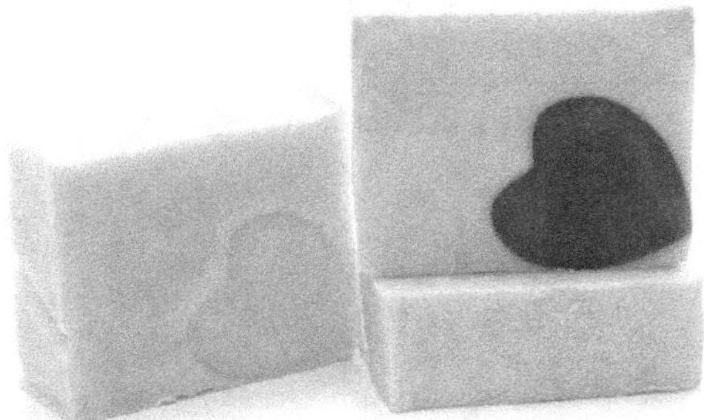

This method is a take on the Swedish Egg White Soap that is famed for keeping women's skin soft and smooth during the harsh winter environment. Vitamin E adds antioxidants to the soap to further protect delicate facial skin. The rose water and rose oil are both soothing and refreshing. Yields 15-20 five-ounce bars of soap.

Ingredients:

- 300g palm oil
- 200g coconut oil
- 600g olive oil
- 3 egg whites
- 50g vitamin e oil
- 1 ounce rose essential oil or rose absolute
- 325g rose water
- 161.8g lye

Directions:

1. Follow the instructions for making cold processed soaps.

2. Rose water takes the place of regular distilled water in this recipe.

3. Temper the egg whites with a little warm olive oil so that they do not scramble when added at trace.

4. It is best to not make this soap at a temperature exceeding 120°F/49°C. It will also help keep the integrity of the egg whites.

5. Add the egg whites, vitamin E and rose essential oil at trace.

6. Insulate for twenty-four hours and check every day for hardness. When the soap is firm, remove from the molds and allow to cure for at least two weeks before using.

Summer Lime Bar

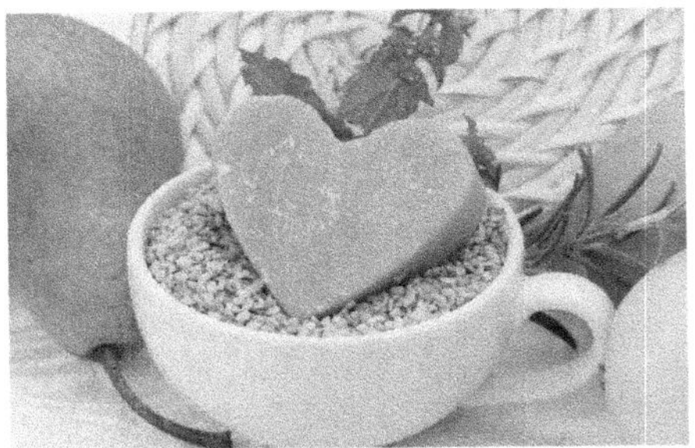

This is a basic vegetable bar recipe with added moisturizers to help repair parched, damaged summer skin. The avocado oil, cocoa butter, and vitamin E help to heal and protect while the lime zest and essential oils provide a soothing and refreshing scent. Yields 15-20 five-ounce bars.

Ingredients:

- 250g coconut oil
- 300g palm oil
- 500g olive oil
- 150g avocado oil
- 100g cocoa butter
- 30g vitamin E
- 2 tablespoons lime zest
- 2 tablespoons dried lavender, ground
- 1-ounce sandalwood essential oil
- 1-ounce cypress essential oil
- 390g distilled water
- 191.5g lye

Directions:

1. Follow the instructions for making cold processed soaps.

2. Add the vitamin E with the main oils.

3. Add the lime zest, dried lavender, and essential oils at trace.

4. Insulate for twenty-four hours and check every day for hardness. When the soap is firm, remove from the molds and allow to cure for at least two weeks before using.

Herbal Shampoo Bar

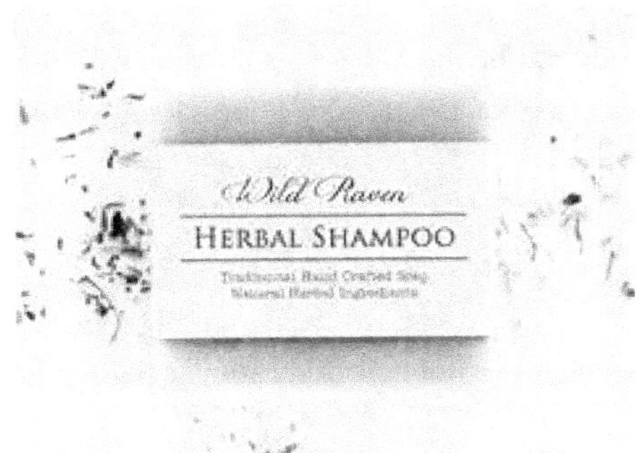

There is another example of how to use one of the basic formulas tc create a specialized soap to suit your needs. The hemp and jojoba oils help to condition the hair. Hops are added for their famed hair beautifying qualities and rosemary helps to soothe an irritated scalp and prevents dry scalp skin. Yields 15-20 five-ounce bars.

Ingredients:

- 250g coconut oil
- 300g palm oil
- 500g olive oil
- 100g hemp seed oil
- 75g jojoba oil
- 1-ounce lavender essential oils
- 1-ounce rosemary essential oil
- 2 tablespoons ground hops
- 360g distilled water
- 176g lye

Directions:

1.   Place the ground hops in a tea ball or infuser and make a tea infusion with the hops and distilled water. Let the hops steep for twenty-four hours. Remove the ground hops from the tea bag and reserve.

2.   Follow the instructions for making cold processed soaps.

3.   Add the reserved ground hops, lavender essential oil, and rosemary essential oil at trace.

4.   Insulate for twenty-four hours and check every day for hardness. When the soap is firm, remove from the molds and allow to cure for at least two weeks before using.

Invigorating Foot Soap

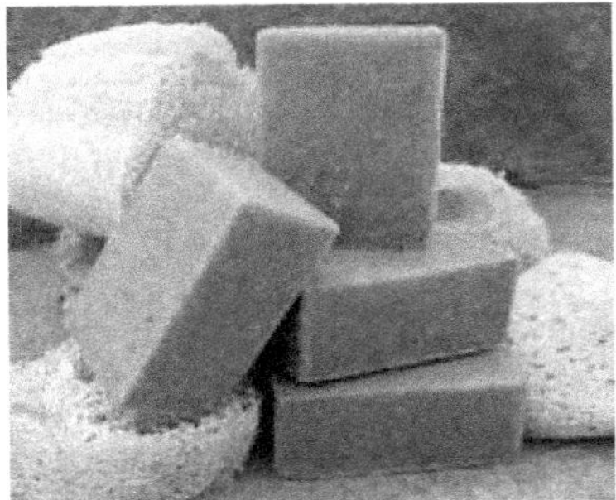

This citrusy soap is mild with a white lather to help soothe the skin. The coffee added provides a gentle exfoliant. This bar will leave your feet soft, smooth and refreshed. Yields 15-20 five-ounce bars of soap.

Ingredients:

- 300g beef tallow
- 150g shea butter
- 50g beeswax
- 400g olive oil
- 100g avocado oil
- 2 tablespoons coarse ground coffee
- 1 teaspoon orange zest
- 1 teaspoon lemon zest
- 1 teaspoon lime zest
- 315g distilled water
- 154.25g lye

Directions:

1. Follow the instructions for making cold processed soaps.

2. Add the ground coffee, orange zest, lemon zest, and lime zest at trace.

3. Insulate for twenty-four hours and check every day for hardness. When the soap is firm, remove from the molds and allow to cure for at least two weeks before using.

Her Shave Soap

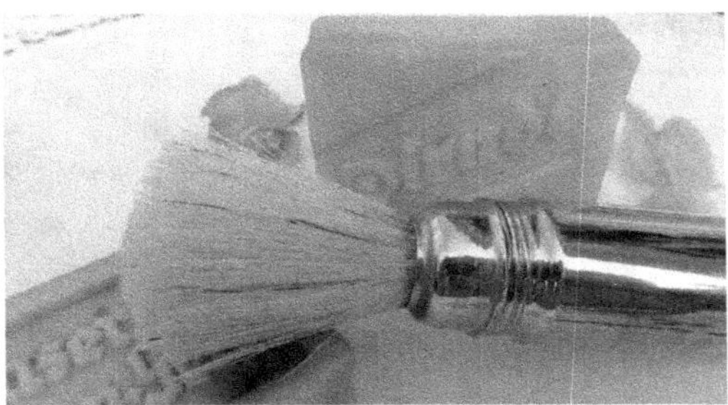

A very mild shave soap that will produce fine, thick and moisturizing lather. The glycerin and honey protect the skin and the clay provides a nice glide for a razor. This soap is mild and conditioning enough to use for daily shaving purposes. Yields 15-20 five-ounce bars of soap.

Ingredients:

- 400g beef tallow
- 400g olive oil
- 75g jojoba oil
- 100g shea butter
- 100g wheat germ oil
- 50g glycerin
- 30g bentonite clay
- 30g honey
- 1-ounce chamomile essential oil
- 1-ounce lavender essential oil
- 330g distilled water
- 163.25g lye

Directions:

1. Follow the instructions for making cold processed soaps.

2. Add the glycerin, bentonite clay, honey, chamomile essential oil, and lavender essential oil at trace.

3. Insulate for twenty-four hours and check every day for hardness. When the soap is firm, remove from the molds and allow to cure for at least two weeks before using.

Old-Fashioned Pine Tar Soap

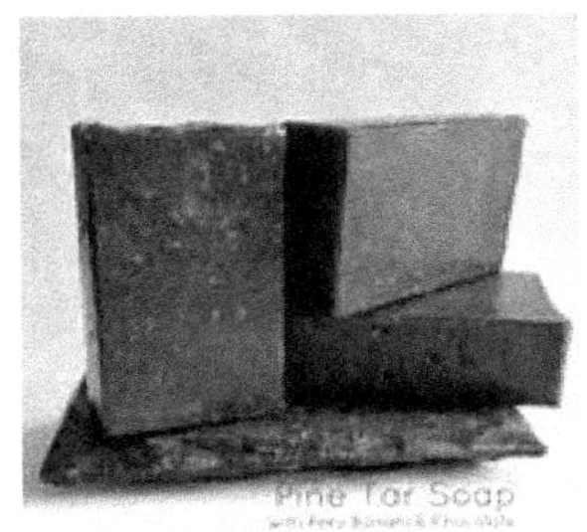

This nostalgic DIY soap is the answer to dry, itchy skin, eczema, dandruff, and psoriasis.

Ingredients:

- 13.5 oz. lard
- 13.5 oz. olive oil
- 8.2 oz. palm kernel oil
- 5.8 oz. sunflower oil
- 7.2 oz. pine tar
- 5.9 oz. lye
- 15.8 oz. water
- 2 oz. lavender, tea tree, eucalyptus, and Siberian fir essential oil blend
- 1 tbsp. sugar added to the water for the lye solution, before you add the lye

Directions:

Follow the Cold Process Soap Making method.

Peppermint and Rosemary Soap

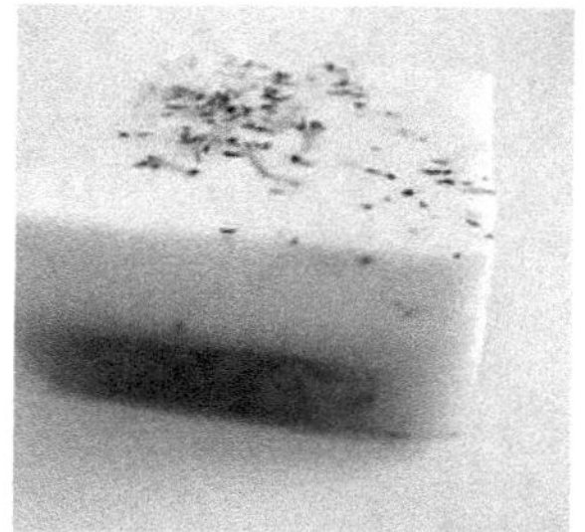

Ingredients:

- 15 oz. olive oil
- 13 oz. coconut oil
- 2.6 oz. castor oil
- 16 oz. distilled water
- 6.2 oz. lye
- 0.8 oz. peppermint essential oil
- 0.8 rosemary essential oil
- 0.4 oz. sage essential oil
- ¼ oz. spirulina
- 1 oz. dried peppermint leaves

Directions:

Follow the Cold Process Soap Making method.

Aloe Vera Soap

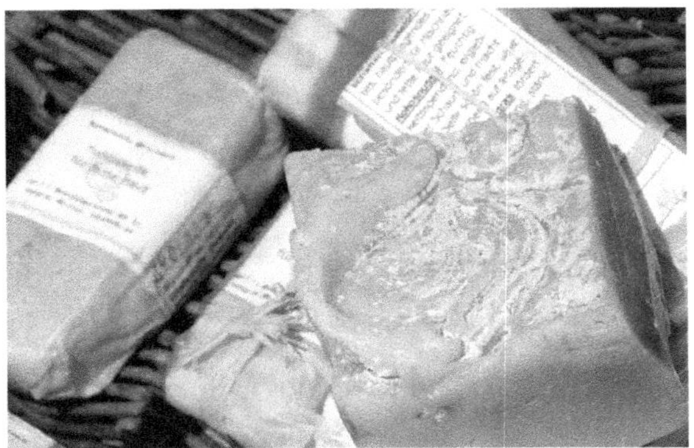

Ingredients:

- 15 oz. refined coconut oil
- 13.5 oz. extra virgin olive oil
- 10.5 oz. lard
- 2.5 oz. organic shea butter
- 10 oz. aloe vera gel and water puree
- 6.5 oz. lye
- 10 oz. purified water

Directions:

Use the Cold Process Soap Making method.

Winter Rose Soap

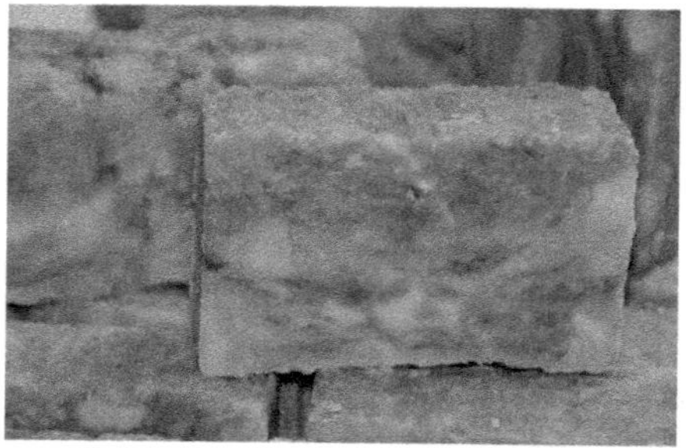

Ingredients:

- 28 oz. refined coconut oil
- 42 oz. extra virgin olive oil
- 12 oz. sunflower oil
- 11.73 oz. Lye
- 26 oz. strained rose petal infusion (create a tea)
- At trace, stir in 1 tablespoon each of rosehip seed oil, jojoba oil and melted shea butter. (optional, makes a higher superfatted bar)
- Also at trace, add a few teaspoons geranium essential oil.

Directions:

Use the Cold Process Soap Making method for this recipe.

Chapter 3 – Melt and Pour Soaps

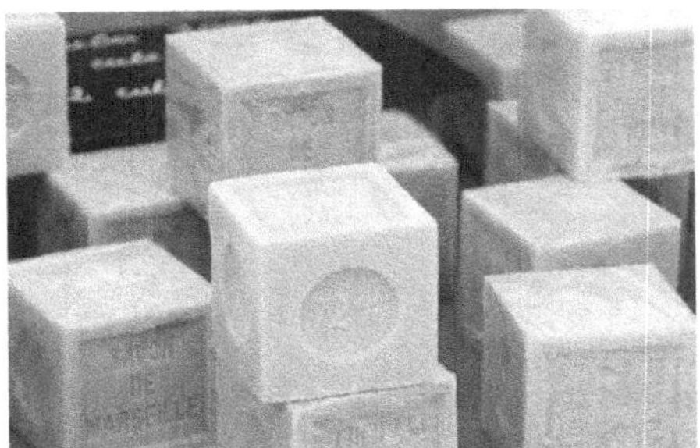

Here you will find some incredibly simple ideas for personalizing melt and pour glycerin soap bases. You will find that these recipes are given in volume measurements rather than the weight measurements used in making cold processed soaps. This is because with melt and pours soap, and you do not depend on a chemical reaction to occur for the soap to form. Therefore, the units of measurement do not need to be as precise. While these recipes inspire you, the reality is that the sky is the limit with melt and pour soaps. Let your imagination run wild.

*As a side note, we have not included any rebatch or hand-milled recipes in this book, as those depend significantly upon what type of soap you are using to rebatch as well as the already existing ingredients. You can modify any of the melt and pour recipes to suit a hand-milled soap as well.

Simple Exfoliating Bar

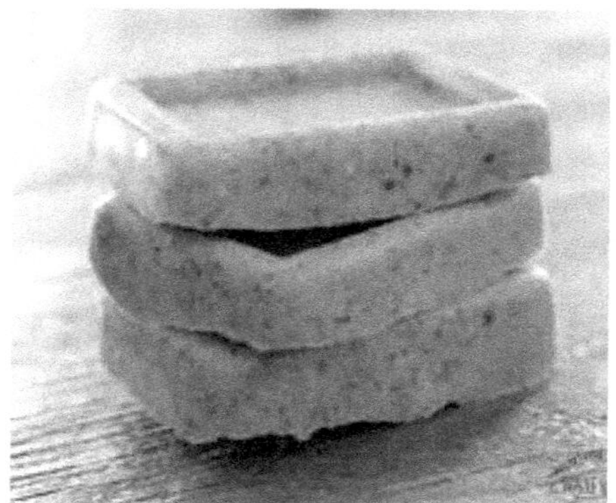

This bar is a perfect example of how you can take a clear melt and pour base and turn it into a customized spa bar. The exfoliants gently brush away dry skin, and the coffee invigorates and conditions. Yields up to four bars, depending on the size and shape of your molds.

Ingredients:

- 2 cups melt and pour soap base, grated
- ½ cup almonds, finely ground
- 2 teaspoons coffee grounds
- 15-20 drops sweet orange essential oil

Directions:

1. Follow the instructions provided for melt and pour soap.

Melt and Pour Tropical Oasis Bar

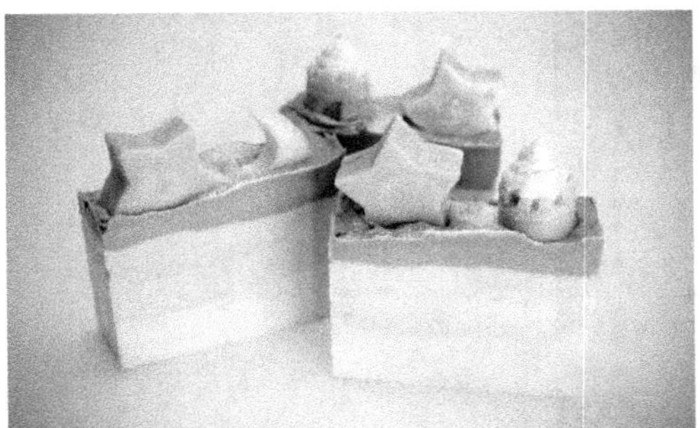

This bar will instantly take you away to the tropical oasis cf your dreams. Laced with coconut, citrus, and jasmine, this makes for the perfect summertime bar. Yields up to four bars, depending upon the size and shape of your molds.

Ingredients:

- 2 cups melt and pour soap base, grated
- ¼ cup almonds, finely ground
- ¼ cup shredded coconut, finely grated
- 1 tablespoon lime zest
- 10 drops lime essential oil
- 5 drops jasmine essential oil

Directions:

1. Follow the instructions provided for melt and pour soap.

Garden Mint Bar

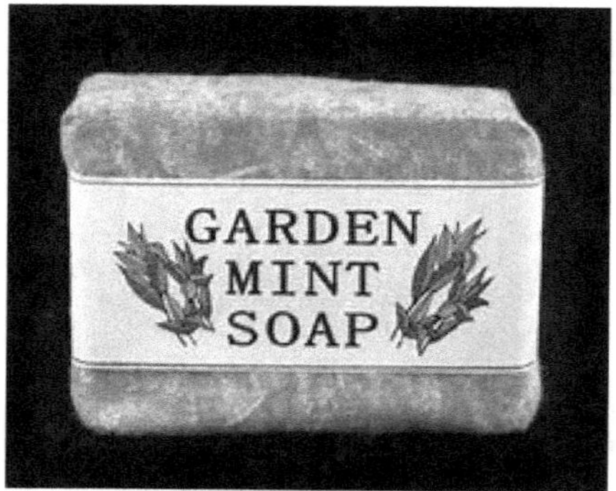

This refreshing mint bar is a perfect reminder of a fresh herb garden. This bar makes a good soap for both warm and cold weather, with the addition of soothing powdered milk. Yields up to four bars, depending upon the size and shape of your molds.

Ingredients:

- 2 cups melt and pour soap base
- ½ cup powdered milk
- ½ cup dried mint leaves, finely ground
- 10 drops peppermint essential oil
- 5 drops rosemary essential oil

Directions:

1. Follow the instructions provided for melt and pour soap.

Chocolate-Covered Fruit Bar

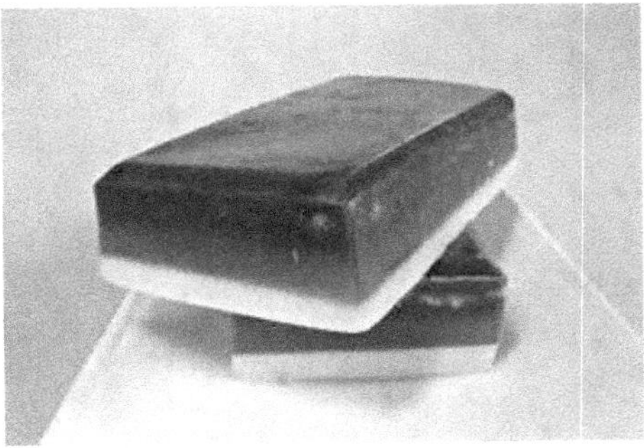

This bar is truly decadent and so mouth-watering that you will need to include instructions not to eat it! Yields up to four bars depending upon the size and shape of your molds.

Ingredients:

- 2 cups melt and pour soap base, grated
- ¼ cup powdered milk
- 1 teaspoon cocoa powder
- 1 tablespoon candied orange peel, chopped.
- 10 drops sweet orange essential oil
- 5 drops peppermint essential oil

Directions:

1. Follow the instructions provided for melt and pour soap.

Spicy Shower Bar

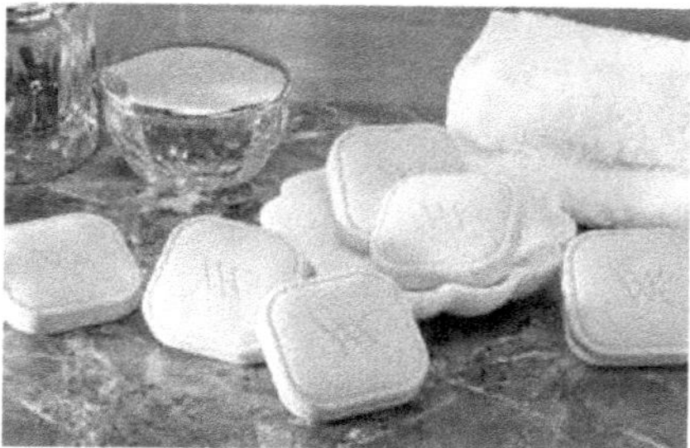

This bar makes a wonderful gift for the men in your life or anyone who prefers a more earthy and spicy smelling soap. The honey and powdered milk are moisturizing, while the herbs are healing and soothing. Yields approximately four bars depending on the size and shape of your molds.

Ingredients:

- 2 cups melt and pour soap base, grated
- ¼ cup powdered milk
- 2 teaspoons honey
- 1 teaspoon ground sage
- 1 teaspoon dried basil
- 2 teaspoons fresh rosemary, ground
- 5 drops cinnamon essential oil
- 10 drops rosemary essential oil

Directions:

1. Follow the instructions provided for melt and pour soap.

Sweet Honey Bar

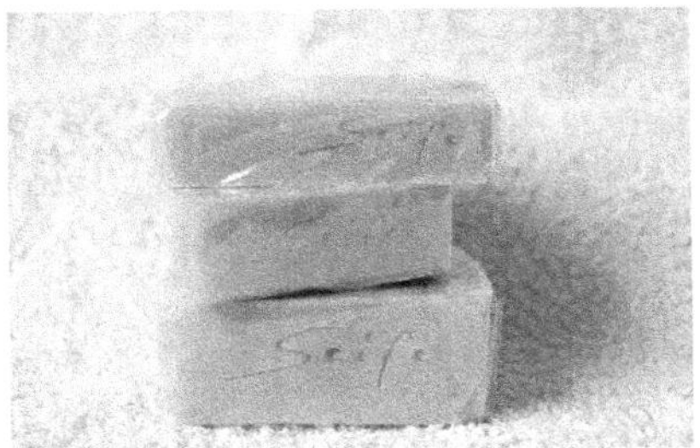

You can add nourishing ingredients such as honey, wheat germ, and oatmeal to your melt and pour soap base to create the soap that looks, feels, and smells like a unique bar. Yields approximately four bars of soap depending on the size and shape of your mold.

Ingredients:

- 2 cups melt and pour soap base
- 2 tablespoons beeswax pellets
- 2 tablespoons honey
- 1 tablespoon wheat germ
- 1 tablespoon oatmeal, finely ground
- 10 drops bergamot essential oil

Directions:

1. Follow the instructions provided for melt and pour soap.

Chapter 4 – Other Soaps

Peppermint and Tea Tree Oil Acne Soap

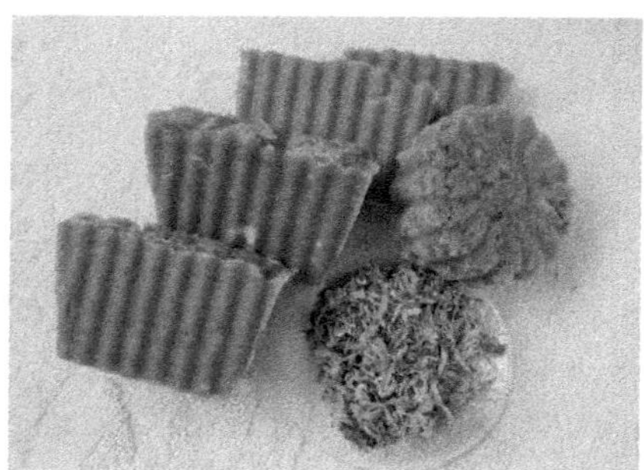

Most over-the-counter acne medicines, cleansers, and soaps are full of strong chemicals. Unfortunately, many people mistake this as being a good thing. They think that they need harsh chemicals to kill their blemishes and that the key to curing acne is to dry out their skin.

This couldn't be further from the truth. In reality, drying your skin makes it produce even more oil, which in turn produces more pimples. Strong chemicals inflame the skin and make it dry and flaky. This acne soap is gentle yet contains natural ingredients that prevent breakouts. Coconut oil is an antibacterial that kills the bacteria in/on your skin that causes acne. Neem oil is also an anti-bacterial and helps reduce redness and inflammation caused by acne. Tea tree oil works as well as prescription drugs like benzoyl peroxide to remedy pimples. Castor oil cleans pores by pulling out excess oils and bacteria. Olive oil is an antioxidant, which helps reduce the appearance of acne scars.

This soap is safe and ready for use after it hardens.

Ingredients:

- Peppermint Essential Oil (1 oz.)
- Tea Tree Oil (1 oz.)
- Lye (4 ½ oz.)
- Water (10 oz.)
- Organic Cold-pressed Olive Oil (10 oz.)
- Organic, Unrefined, Cold-pressed Coconut Oil (10 oz.)
- Organic Castor Oil (2 oz.)
- Organic Palm Oil (3 oz.)
- Organic Neem Oil (6 oz.)
- Beeswax (2 oz.)

Directions:

1. Pour water into a large stainless steel or glass bowl.

2. Pour lye into water, stirring it until the lye has dissolved.

3. Fill a large bowl halfway with cold water and ice cubes. Place the bowl with water and lye into this larger bowl. Make sure that the water and lye mixture stays cold. If the ice melts, add more.

4. Pour beeswax and olive oil, coconut oil, castor oil, palm oil, and neem oil into a pot. Heat them on medium-low heat on the stove until they've all melted.

5. Transfer the beeswax and oil mixture into a crockpot. Heat on the lowest setting.

6.   Slowly pour the lye and water into the crockpot. Stir until well mixed.

7.   Use the stick blender to blend the mixture in the crockpot. Blend for three to five minutes. By then it should reach trace.

8.   Place the lid on the crockpot and leave the mixture covered for at least one hour while on lowest heat setting. The mixture should look a bit translucent.

9.   Add peppermint oil and tea tree oil to the mixture.

10.   Pour mixture into soap molds.

11.   After 24 hours, remove from the molds and cut it into bars. If they're still not completely hard, leave them uncovered for a few hours.

Neem Oil Soap for Psoriasis

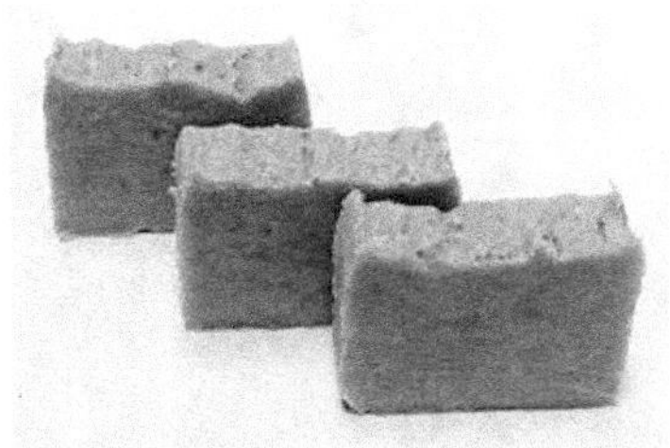

Psoriasis flare-ups can be very painful. Many people feel embarrassed of the dry red patches that populate their skin during a psoriasis outbreak. Neem oil has been used to clear up the patches brought up by psoriasis. Because it's an emollient, neem oil can soften the scaly, dry patches of skin caused by a psoriasis flare-up. It also soothes the itchiness and can reduce redness. Try this soap if you have psoriasis and are in need of soothing an outbreak.

Ingredients:

- Organic Neem Oil (3 ½ oz.)
- Lye (4 $\frac{9}{10}$ oz.)
- Distilled Water (12 oz.)
- Organic Argan Oil (1 $\frac{3}{10}$ oz.)
- Organic, Unrefined, Cold-pressed Coconut Oil (3⅗ oz.)
- OrganicCold-pressed Olive Oil (4⅗ oz.)
- Organic Apricot Kernel Oil (3⅗ oz.)
- Organic Tamanu Oil (1 oz.)
- Organic Wheat Germ Oil (1 $\frac{3}{10}$ oz.)

- Organic Cocoa Butter (1 ³⁄₁₀ oz.)
- Organic Grape Seed Oil (10⅘ oz.)
- Organic Shea Butter (1 ³⁄₁₀ oz.)
- Organic Palm Kernel Flakes (7⅕ oz.)

Directions:

1. Pour water into a large stainless steel or glass bowl.

2. Pour lye into water, stirring it until the lye has dissolved.

3. Fill a large bowl halfway with cold water and ice cubes. Place the bowl with water and lye into this larger bowl. Make sure that the water and lye mixture stays cold. If the ice melts, add more.

4. Pour the cocoa butter, shea butter, and the argan oil, coconut oil, olive oil, apricot kernel oil, tamanu oil, wheat germ oil, and palm kernel flakes into the non-aluminum pot. Heat them on the stove on medium heat. Once everything has melted, take the pot off of the stove. Set it aside and leave it to cool down.

5. Allow the butter and oil mixture and the water and lye mixture to cool down until they're between 110 and 115 degrees Fahrenheit.

6. Pour the water and lye into the butter and oil mixture. Blend with a stick blender until it begins to thicken and reaches trace.

7.   Pour the neem oil into the mixture. Stir it in until it's well blended.

8.   Pour the mixture into soap mold. Cover the mold and let it sit for at least 24 hours.

9.   Remove soap from the mold and cut it into bars. Let the bars cure for a minimum of three weeks.

Winter Foot Soap Soak

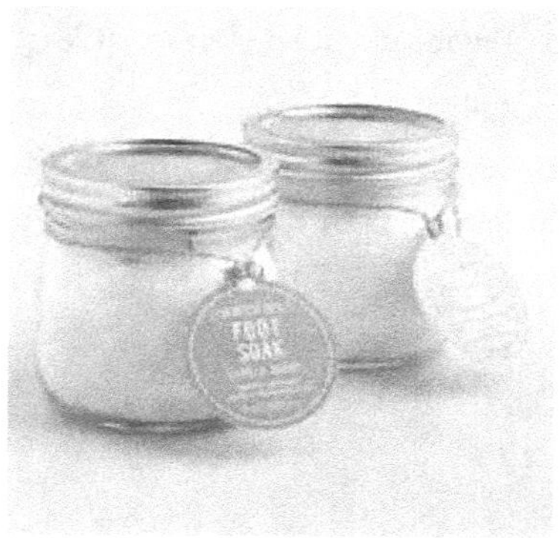

When your feet are feeling frigid due to plummeting winter temperatures, this sudsy DIY foot soak is sure to warm them up.

Ingredients:

- ¼ c. lemon juice
- ¼ c. milk
- 3 tbsps. extra virgin olive oil
- 1 tbsp. castile soap
- 1/8 tsp. cinnamon

Directions:

Place all ingredients in a large basin and add hot warm. Give the solution a stir with your hand, and allow your feet to soak for as long as you like.

Happy Winter Skin Facial Soap

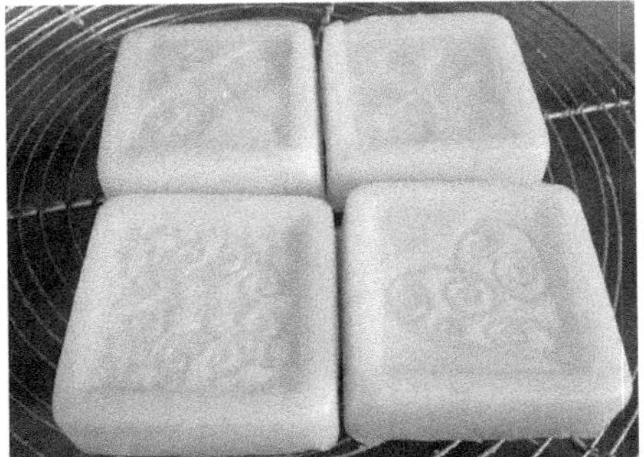

Is your face dried out due to frosty winter air? Treat yourself to this moisture-rich facial soap.

Ingredients:

- 2 apple slices, peeled
- ½ c. plain yogurt
- ½ c. tbsp. olive oil
- ½ tbsp. raw honey

Directions:

Blend all ingredients in a food processor or blender until smooth and creamy. Massage soap onto skin and allow to sit for 5-minutes. Rinse with warm water.

Moisturizing Honey Shower Wash

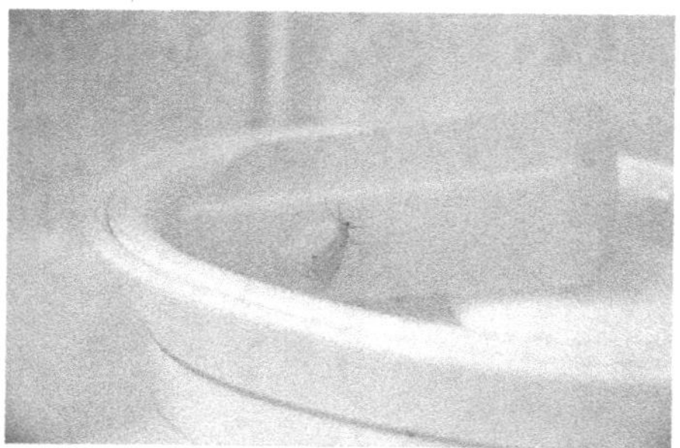

Ingredients:

- 2/3 c. castile soap
- ¼ c. raw honey
- 2 tbsp. grapeseed oil
- 1 tsp. vitamin E oil
- 50 – 60 drops vanilla essential oil

Directions:

Place all ingredients in a recycled shampoo or body wash container and shake vigorously. Squirt onto a washcloth or loofah.

Homemade Dish Soap

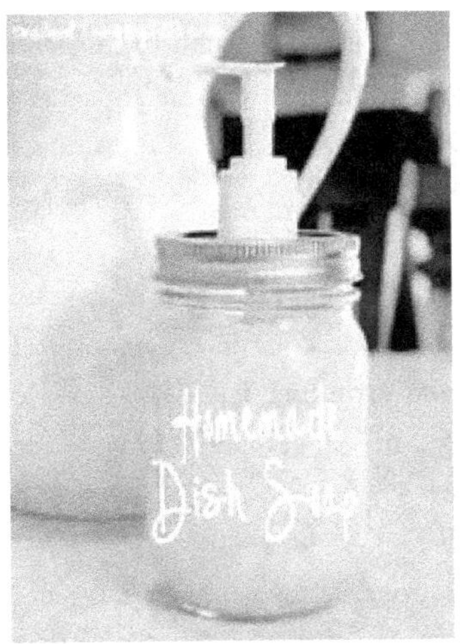

Ingredients:

- 1 ¾ c. boiling water
- 1 tbsp. borax
- 1 tbsp. grated Ivory or Castile bar soap
- 15 – 20 drops of orange or lemon essential oil

Directions:

Heat water until boiling. Next, add the borax and grated bar soap to a medium bowl. Then, pour the boiled water over the top of the soap mixture. Whisk until the soap dissolves. Allow the mixture to cool for about 8 hours, stirring now and then. Transfer the dish soap to a squirt bottle and add in the essential oil. Shake well to combine.

Conclusion

Washing your body shouldn't be treated as a chore. Instead, it should be treated as a ritual. You should find enjoyment, satisfaction, and pleasure in bathing. Take the time to really feel the textures of these unique soaps on your skin. Slow down and deeply inhale their aromas.

Your body is special and important. Washing with homemade organic soap is so much better for your skin, mind and spirit than using a commercial soap! You deserve so much more than artificial fragrances and toxic chemicals. You deserve nourishing ingredients that soothe the skin, delight the senses, and stimulate the mind.

Now that you see the positive effect that natural soaps can have on your skin, you should continue your soap education. Research new fragrances and additives that you can put in your soap. Think hard about what feelings you want to evoke when you shower. Think hard about what your skin needs. Does it need more moisture? Do you have a rash? Learn about more ingredients that can repair your skin.

Continue to think about the ingredients in your soap, and also in the environment around you. Read labels, ask questions. Is this good for me? Is there a harmful ingredient in this?

Now that you know that soap making is a fun, fulfilling activity, we hope that you continue to make soaps for yourselves and for the people you love. Share your creations with others. Tell them to take a long shower with one of your soaps and ask them if they notice a difference in their skin, body, mind, and spirit.